Living In Color

Living In Color

Renae Knapp

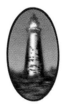

Lighthouse Publishing Group, Inc.
Seattle, Washington

Lighthouse Publishing Group, Inc.
© 1998 Renae Knapp

Library of Congress Catalog-in-Publications Data
Knapp, Renae
Living in color/Renae Knapp
p. cm.
ISBN 0-910019-75-4
1. Color--Psychological aspects. I. Title.
BF789.C7K53   1998
152.14'5--dc21   98-22594 CIP

Lighthouse Publishing Group, Inc. would like to thank the following people for their invaluable help, without which *Living In Color* would not be possible:

Executive Director: Cheryle Hamilton
Production and Promotion Director: Alison Curtis
Art Director: Mark Engelbrecht
Book Designer: Judy Burkhalter
Cover Designer: Angela Wilson
Main Photographer: Zachary A. Cherry
Secondary Photographers: Jason Norris, Vaughn Tanner, Robert Dorr, Hoya Corporation, Renae Knapp Color Institute Salons, Roy Pryor, Vision Industry Council of America, Mirror Image
Cover Photographer: Bill Pegram
Make-up Artist: Julie Mitchell
Make-up Assistants: Jerry and Andrea Miller, Noel Thomas, Karen Larsen
Editors and Proofers: Jill Kramer, Linda Johns, Vicki VanHise, Connie Suehiro, Bethany McVannel, Jason Norris, Sam Hemenway, Cynthia Fliege, and Randy Knapp

Note: Every effort has been made to accurately reproduce all of the colors, color palettes, and color samples in this book. However, due to the limitations inherent in the color printing process, discrepancies may occur. Therefore, the colors and samples in this book are meant only as a guideline. For the most accurate color guide, please use a Renae Knapp "Color Pro" Fan Deck. For ordering information call 1-888-395-9323 or visit www.livingincolor.com.

The Blue Base/Yellow Base Color System®, Renae Knapp Color Institute™, Spectrum 1 Colors™, and Spectrum 2 Colors™ are registered trademarks of Renae Knapp Color Institute Salons.

The Color Personality Reference Questionnaire was researched and developed by Keith Rogers, Ph.D., Brigham Young University and printed by permission of Renae Knapp Color Institute Salons Publishing Group, Inc.

Published by Lighthouse Publishing Group, Inc.
14675 Interurban Avenue South
Seattle, Washington 98168-4664
1-800-706-8657
(206) 901-3100 fax
www.lighthousebooks.com

Printed in Canada
10 9 8 7 6 5 4 3 2 1

Other Books By Lighthouse Publishing Group, Inc.

Wealth 101, Wade Cook

Brilliant Deductions, Wade Cook

The Secret Millionaire Guide To Nevada Corporations, John Childers, Jr.

Million Heirs, John Childers, Jr.

Bear Market Baloney, Wade Cook

Blueprints For Success, Volume 1, Various Authors

On Track Investing, David Hebert

Rolling Stocks, Gregory Witt

Sleeping Like A Baby, John Hudelson

Stock Market Miracles, Wade Cook

Wall Street Money Machine, Wade Cook

101 Ways To Buy Real Estate Without Cash, Wade Cook

Cook's Book On Creative Real Estate, Wade Cook

How To Pick Up Foreclosures, Wade Cook

Owner Financing, Wade Cook

Real Estate Money Machine, Wade Cook

Real Estate For Real People, Wade Cook

A+, Wade Cook

Business Buy The Bible, Wade Cook

Don't Set Goals, Wade Cook

Wade Cook's Power Quotes, Wade Cook

Contents

This book is dedicated to people everywhere
who are devoted to peace, harmony,
and balance in their lives—
you are a constant source of inspiration to me—
along with my husband, Clive,
a Spectrum 2, and our five sons,
Barry, Michael, Danny, David, and Rich,
three Spectrum 2's and two Spectrum 1's,
who literally live life in color with me.
I love you very much!

Acknowledgments

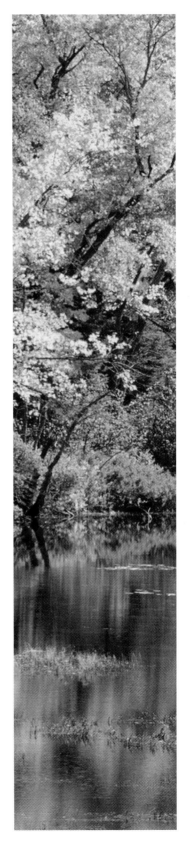

Thank you first of all to the models in this book. Although not professional models, they have beautifully demonstrated how the Blue Base/Yellow Base Color System works for anyone in their everyday life.

Barry Knapp, thank you for helping establish the vision and operations of Renae Knapp Color Institute Salons around the world.

Randy Knapp, RKCIS Corporate Editor, you keep us committed to details and excellence.

Roy Pryor, RKCIS Corporate Photographer, your professionalism is appreciated.

Cheryle Hamilton, thank you for vision and total creativity in making this book a reality.

Alison Curtis, thank you for taking this project to a new level of quality from beginning to end.

Steve Wirrick, thank you for believing in this project.

Julie Mitchell, RKCIS Seattle, your tireless efforts handling photo shoots and doing make-up was invaluable. Thank you, Julie, we couldn't have done it without you.

Masako Post, RKCIS Corporate Executive Japanese Affairs, whose efforts, support, and help is endless in coordinating RKCIS U.S. with RKCIS Japan.

Tracy Utterbach, RKCIS Corporate Executive with our Institute Salon Division. Thank you for your generous help setting up our Salons.

Sadako Kashikura, thank you for teaching the system in Japan with such great integrity and loyalty.

Spectrum 2, Japan, thank you to all of the distributors and image consultants for their continuing loyalty and teaching the science of the system in Japan.

Keiko Shimojyu, Hoya Corporation, Japan, thank you for having the vision, promoting so beautifully the system throughout the optical industry, and taking the system to the highest level in Japan.

OCA, Optical Color Analysis, Japan, thank you to all of the members for teaching and promoting the system in the Optical Industry in Japan.

Toshiko Suzuki, thank you for your continued support and love of the system in Japan.

Carol Norbeck, my lifelong friend, thank you for helping arrange pictures and giving valuable input from the optical industry in the U.S.

VICA, Vision Industry Council of America, thank you for the pictures and support.

Panasonic of Japan, Pana Homes, thank you for creating beautiful, harmonious interiors in Japan.

Bob Bush, Ph.D., thank you for your vision and help at Northwest Missouri State University.

Dianne Knapp, thank you for tireless and endless time, efforts, and ingenious creativity and graphics. RKCIS would not be a company without you.

David Knapp, thank you for your constant loyalty and devotion to keeping RKCIS moving forward.

Rayolla Mitchell, thank you for the use of your beautiful home.

Scott Conover, thank you for the continuing technical support.

Jeff Kunz, thank you for your vision of how to implement the system in technology.

I also want to thank the following people for valuable feedback: Darrell Utterbach, Lori Prokop, Abi Carmen, Julie and Dennis Farr, Sally and Don Cox, Bonnie Knell, Mary Wellmon, Lynnette Michael, David Hanen, Marilla Hamor, Ray Linford, Danny Knapp, Ted Lindauer, James Thompson, Arnold and Frances Knapp, Saundra Labatto, Gwena and Melvin Fish, Naomi Silveira, Cindy Catlin, Ken and Elnora Mason, Connie Loosli, Lyman and Karrie Nielson, Lin Na Lin, and Jim Diver.

Preface

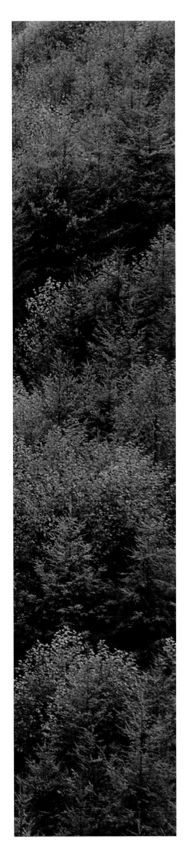

What would you think if I told you there was a way you could wear purple or yellow or black—or any color you thought you couldn't wear—and look good? How would you feel if I showed you how to analyze your wardrobe and make-up, then correct it, all in a matter of minutes, by yourself, without the aid of expensive experts? Or, what if I could give you something that would guarantee you'd never make another costly mistake at the bargain counter or (what's worse) the couturier?

The Blue Base/Yellow Base Color System is an unbelievably simple tool that completely solves any color problems you may have—and with it, your whole problem with how you "look." Whether it's your make-up, eyeglasses, hair, clothes, home, or even mood, the Blue Base/Yellow Base Color System can bring them into beautiful harmony. From now on, you can really look dynamic all the way, all the time.

I know this sounds like an extravagant claim, and I am among the most skeptical of people. However, I made this claim in my first best selling book, *Beyond The Color Explosion,* and people everywhere reacted the same way I did when I first heard about the Blue Base/Yellow Base Color System. They were saying things like "I don't believe it!" "How come I haven't heard of this before?" and "What were we waiting for?"

First, believe it! Blue Base/Yellow Base is real: it works. It's the only color system to have been thoroughly tested; through seven university studies (including some at California

Polytechnic and Stanford), through 40 years of practical use, through refinement by professionals in the textile, cosmetics, and building industries, even through science itself.

Second, *that's why you haven't heard of it.* The Blue Base/Yellow Base Color System has been a behind the scenes professional tool—like those tricks models have used for years—that is only now filtering down to working men and women seeking all day glamour. Before now, you could learn the Blue Base/Yellow Base Color System in textbooks, industry manuals, and company meetings, but that was about it.

I first heard of Blue Base/Yellow Base years ago in Southern California when I was spokesperson for a top cosmetics company. I was attending a seminar when a packet of Blue and Yellow Base color samples came into my hands. I immediately saw its possibilities! Though I worked with color every day and had access to all the color techniques and systems, those techniques were never really usable on the spot. When helping people with make-up or clothing choices, I always seemed to wind up relying on my eye and experience. There was no way I could send my experience home with anyone. I could only tell people what to do and wear, not teach people why and how. With Blue Base/Yellow Base, I saw something portable, workable, manageable, and filled with opportunity. I knew the difference the right colors could make, and I saw Blue Base/Yellow Base as a real gift.

To find out more, I tracked down Robert Dorr, the man who discovered the Blue Base/Yellow Base Color System, and who happened to live in a nearby suburb. I began to work with him on the Blue Base/Yellow Base Color System. Bob Dorr became my mentor.

Since then, I have been using, adapting, teaching, and perfecting the system, all while conducting further research and studies into this amazing science of color. I have heard literally thousands of stories from around the world about how the Blue Base/Yellow Base Color System has changed people's

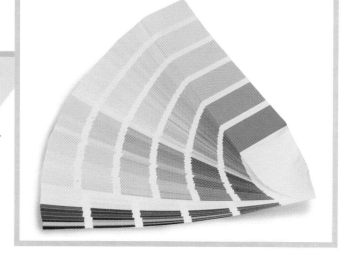

Renae Knapp created Blue Base and Yellow Base "Personal Color Pro" Fan Decks to assist you with your color selection. These fans are portable, easy to use guides for choosing the right colors and are available by calling 1-888-395-9323.

lives. My classes and lectures ring with exclamations such as "I don't believe it!" and "This really works!" However, the most wonderful statements all begin with "This has changed my life."

This was an exciting time for me. I was busy doing what I loved: analyzing and discovering people's personal colors and helping them improve their image. I was busy redressing them to take them from "not so credible" to "very credible," helping them find new levels of income and self-esteem. I was showing average women how to be above average by discovering the power hidden within themselves through the acquired knowledge of who they were in the color spectrum. It was exhilarating and euphoric to watch lives turn completely around as financial, personal, and spiritual rewards abounded throughout lives—all because of the knowledge I taught them through color! I saw the power harmonious color had over self-doubt and intimidation. I saw how knowledge of color harmony created power within the individual. I knew for sure the Blue Base/Yellow Base Color System worked.

My life at that time was very hectic. I was writing my first book on the subject, *Beyond The Color Explosion*. I wanted everyone on the planet to have access to the powerful knowledge behind color science. I felt that everyone should know and understand the role that color had in the creation of the planet. My role was to help people add this wonderful knowledge to their lives—I felt like a missionary.

In 1984, I began my first of many incredible experiences working in Japan. The people I met accepted the knowledge I brought about color as a sacred gift that would turn the course of their lives around. They couldn't get enough of the knowledge that I brought to them. They would wait patiently as I discovered each person's colors and analyzed the uniqueness of individual features. Tears of joy and acceptance would run down their faces as they thanked me for teaching them the Blue Base/Yellow Base Color System.

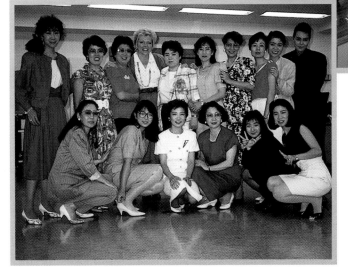

The Blue Base/Yellow Base Color System is easy to use. With only a little training, people learn how to work the system on their own. These photographs were taken at Hoya Optical in Japan, where Japanese Optical Color Analysis professionals (OCA) learn how to work with the Color System and do personal color.

One experience was especially meaningful to me. Since it was my first trip to Japan, many people were anxious for me to experience the beauty and culture of their great country. One day, the vice president of Polaroid Cameras was assigned the task of showing me around. On that day, he took me to a temple site near Osaka and walked me up to a balcony that overlooked a beautiful, lush green garden area. "Look, Renae," he told me, pointing to the garden, "I used to come here as a child. It is one of my favorite spots. I would look over this beautiful hillside and know it was so perfect in the harmony and balance that it reflected. It wasn't until you brought this valuable color science to Japan that I understood why. Now I know. Thank you for bringing this knowledge to Japan."

I was so moved and touched as I stood there and looked at this sacred place, realizing that color had played such an important part in his life. He understood that man should not take the natural harmony of the world and rearrange it or try to reinvent it. Instead, we should look at it, understand it, implement it, and feel the peace it gives us in its silent, powerful way. Learn the gifts color brings and reap the benefits; use them wisely and intelligently. I was humbled and grateful to play even a small part in giving a gift of knowledge to another that could so dramatically affect his life.

One by one, individual by individual, I was learning what a powerful tool the Blue Base/Yellow Base Color System was. It could create harmony and peace in individuals' lives. During this time, I was gathering more and more valuable data about personal coloring, personality traits, and buying habits of the individual. What I was learning was fast becoming the new standard for marketing success in the 21st century.

I learned that individual buying habits could definitely be monitored based on which spectrum the customers were (See Chapter 5). Inventory could actually be purchased based on bottom-line information on what percent of clientele were Blue Base or Yellow Base. Businesses that used my training

Nature is either Blue Base or Yellow Base. Both exist equally. The statue on the right is surrounded by Yellow Base trees. The hillside above is covered with Blue Base trees.

found themselves amazingly accurate on inventory control and purchasing. Referrals to their businesses increased dramatically. Shizue Yonezawa, the owner of over 200 optical shops throughout Japan told me her sales had increased 100% since using the Blue Base/Yellow Base Color System. I loved this feedback so much that I asked her to repeat it to me several times. Each time she bowed and said, "Yes, that is absolutely correct." Wow! As business after business, company after company, and individual after individual kept giving me this feedback, I realized that anyone who was serious about what they did in their business would have to know about this simple, yet amazingly effective, color system.

During this exciting time, I was listed for eight consecutive years in *Who's Who In America* for the Young Presidents Organization's most sought-after and effective speakers. This created a lot of excitement in the corporate arena. I had the opportunity to travel throughout the United States and work in every aspect of the marketplace. With each new experience, my validation of the Blue Base/Yellow Base Color System continued to grow. Over a ten-year period, I worked with thousands of small businesses and large corporations, and over 30,000 individuals of all cultures throughout the world. My findings were consistent and phenomenal. With rare exception, the Blue Base/Yellow Base Color System proved accurate. It never failed. Corporate sales always increased, usage always went up, and lives were always changed through the use of the Blue Base/ Yellow Base Color System.

Most important, the question of *why* was always answered. Why can't I sell these goods? Why don't I like my car? Why don't we use a certain room in the house very much? Why do my patients feel more agitated in this examination room than in the others? Why do I feel more powerful and in control when I wear this certain outfit? Why do I receive better treatment from my clients when I wear certain colors? Why do I like to eat at a certain restaurant? Why does my husband or wife have such bad taste? The answer to these why

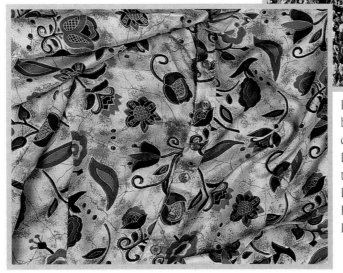

Businesses who purchase inventory based on the percentile of their clients who are Blue Based or Yellow Based have incredibly accurate stock to sales ratios. For example, the Blue Base skirt above would sell better to a Blue Base clientele than the Yellow Base blouse left would.

questions became a very important common denominator everywhere I taught the Blue Base/Yellow Base Color System.

On one occasion, the president of Northwest Missouri State University heard me speak and immediately hired me to fly back to the University to help him with planning the new cultural arts center, library, and snack bar. All things considered, the new projects amounted to millions of dollars in expenses. The *why* in the equation was, "Why can't anyone on the school committee, the architect firm, or the designer agree on anything?" The project was going very slowly as meeting after meeting and decision after decision brought nothing but negative feedback to the President of the University. No one was able to agree on the colors. The designer, in her frustration, tried to cater to everyone's tastes. The architect was beside himself as he purchased $50,000 worth of carpet, only to be met with a school committee that totally disapproved of the choice and the direction the project was going.

These rooms are perfect examples of Yellow Base interiors. A Blue Base person would probably prefer Blue Base rooms, but would still feel the natural harmony and peace of these rooms.

I entered the project as the odd woman out. "Why do we need a color consultant?" seemed to be the general response. The President introduced me to the committee, the architectural firm, and the designer, simply saying, "Do what she tells you to do or you're fired." He then excused himself to run the school, telling me to get back to him with my progress. He gave me a week to unravel the mess.

I first met with the school committee which was composed of university staff and professors. I taught them the Blue Base/Yellow Base Color System. They did what everyone else does when they hear the system for the first time: they went insane with excitement! It put an end to the confusion and it gave them a working tool. It not only took away the guesswork, but also quantified and qualified each step of what they were doing. From a University perspective, it added science, knowledge, and objectivity to a creative, subjective, personal opinion area. It eliminated the concept of "my creative eye is better than your creative eye." There is no such thing. All we had to do was focus on scientifically proven color principles to achieve the necessary harmony and balance.

Next, I met with the interior designer. She was easy to work with because she was at her wits end trying to bring everyone to her side, getting them to like what she was doing. As she learned the Blue Base/Yellow Base Color System and we studied the project together, we discovered that she was a Spectrum 2 (a Yellow Base person). Most of the University committee assigned to the project were Spectrum 1 (Blue Base people). The architect was definitely Blue Base. This was valuable information because now the designer could immediately understand why her choices were considered to be in "bad taste." As we progressed through the week, we carefully and meticulously worked with the purchases that could not be sent back. We concentrated on making the environment around them harmonious. Chairs, tables, and file cabinets were all brought into focus with the environment. Woods were carefully chosen to harmonize with the selected spectrum of each room.

At the end of the week, a meeting was planned with all of the people involved, including the President. Everyone wanted to see the end results from using the color science. Anticipation was high. Several committee members were very nervous that an agreement still would not be reached. Finally, the big day arrived and we gathered around a large table with the President at the head. On one side sat the school committee in charge of the project, while on the other sat the architect and the designer. As I

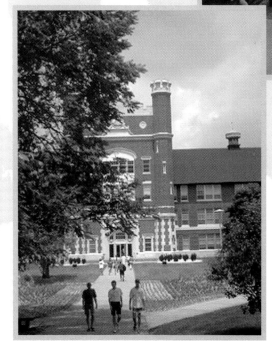

As you can see, the Northwest Missouri State University is a beautiful facility. Bringing balance through color harmony makes the campus appealing and relaxing.

unfolded the plan I had helped put together, each person got more and more excited. Eyes opened wide, and smiles crossed each face as they unanimously agreed that this new plan was perfect! It felt and looked so good!

The most amazing aspect of the whole experience at the Northwest Missouri State University was that the final plans were not much different than what had already been put together before I arrived. The big difference was the removal of mixed spectrums. The new design was now 100% harmonious and free of discord. I had focused the project, much like focusing a camera, by applying the Blue Base/Yellow Base Color System. The rooms were now perfect instead of being a little "off." They didn't assault the nervous system any longer; instead they subtly yet powerfully sent electromagnetic wave lengths through the brain that said, "This feels good. I love it."

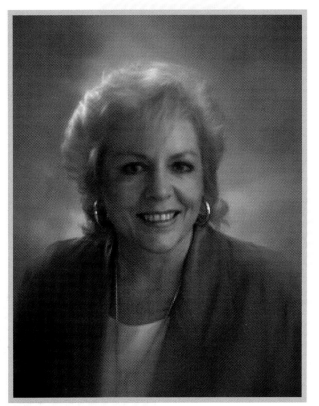

Six months later, I received my real pay in the mail. It was a letter from Bob Bush, Ph.D., the President of Northwest Missouri State University, telling me how he couldn't thank me enough. He said that usage of the remodeled library had gone up 75% and sales in the redone cafeteria had gone up 95%! The cultural arts center was simply loved.

After over two decades of research, I'm happy to offer the Blue Base/Yellow Base Color System to you. It is my hope that learning the Blue Base/Yellow Base Color System will help bring more beauty and harmony to your life. The Blue Base/Yellow Base Color System can become a tool to help you achieve what you want.

Renee Knapp

Introduction

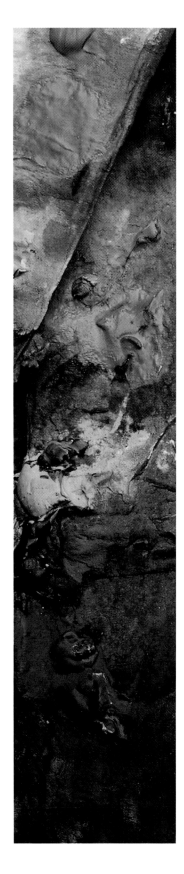

When Robert Dorr first began his research on the Blue Base/Yellow Base Color System, he quickly realized the enormity of what he had discovered. Then, in the 1950s, Stanford University and General Electric certified the Blue Base/Yellow Base Color System one of only three color systems ever proven to be 100% accurate. 100%! To me, that is amazing. Few things are 100% accurate.

When I first taught the Blue Base/Yellow Base Color System in Japan over 12 years ago, Tokyo University researchers also came to the same conclusion. Because of this, the Blue Base/Yellow Base Color System is now taught in many schools throughout Japan. Ongoing research conducted at Renae Knapp Color Institute Salons also reaffirms the validity of the Blue Base/Yellow Base Color System and sheds new light on what you are reading about in this book.

Color Confusion

Unfortunately, some people have taken the simple, 100% accurate, method of Blue Base/Yellow Base colors and complicated it. They have changed the simple fundamentals of the science, and created confusion in the marketplace. As a result, various terms and methods of working with color have sprung up that almost make your eyes roll back in your head.

Several years ago, I received a phone call from a woman who wanted some advice on what to wear to a certain formal occasion. Since I had never seen her before, I asked her to come in and see me. When I saw her, I instantly knew that something was wrong, even though everything appeared to be right.

I asked her if she was happy with the dress she had on. She wasn't sure. Next, I looked into the iris of her eyes and immediately knew that her hair color and make-up were all wrong for her. She told me that she had paid $500 to have her colors done and was informed that she was a "Summer." Armed with this knowledge, and a selection of color swatches, she had thrown out everything in her closet. Then she went out to buy a new wardrobe for her "Summer" look—even though she wasn't sure that she liked the colors or even knew what "Summer" meant.

I hated to inform her that most of the colors she received were wrong for her (even though she instinctively already knew that), and that she was really wearing some of the worst colors possible for her own credibility and self-esteem. The worst part, however, was the simple fact that the colors given to her as a "Summer" created a mixed Spectrum look.

Kiman, a Yellow Base corporate attorney looks hard and made-up in Blue Base colors (above). When she wears Yellow Base colors, she looks natural and trustworthy. Knowledge of your correct color base is vital to enhance and project your natural qualities.

As I taught her the Blue Base/Yellow Base Color System, hope came to her eyes. She could now understand why she was not happy with how she looked. Even better, she now knew *how* to fix it. By the time she left, she was educated with a proven color science she could use on her own!

Change Your Life With Color

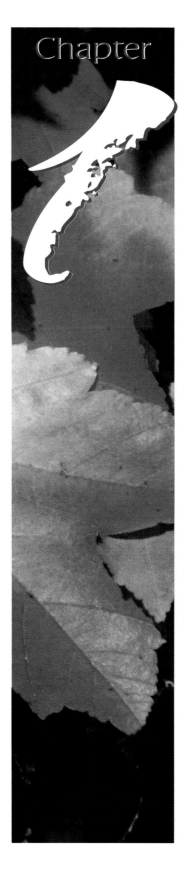

Color has a mystery and magic all its own. Science has proven that color has the first initial impact on our senses. We see color before form. Color influences our emotions and how we feel. We feel peaceful when surrounded by blue. We feel sophisticated and svelte when dressed in black. Our eyes are attracted to red or orange in product labeling or packaging and we are seduced into making a purchase. An atmosphere can seem warm and friendly, or cold and inhospitable, all because of its color.

Our first and successive impressions of color are powerful, even though we are often unconscious of its impact. Color assaults our senses every moment of the day and is subtly linked to our emotions and mental well being. We do not choose to let color affect us; it boldly and consistently intertwines itself with our lives, and gives us a sense of either harmony and peace or confusion and frustration.

Color, like music, must be harmonious. To achieve visual harmony, balance, and proportion, we must harness color's power. This is the secret of the Blue Base/Yellow Base Color System. Understanding Blue Base/Yellow Base colors allows us to surround ourselves with color harmony and peace.

Everyone Has It!

I once overheard a conversation between a customer and the owner of a business that caters weddings. The customer asked, "How do you know what colors to put with other colors?" The owner leaned over close to the woman and said, "Ma'am, you either have it, or you don't." The blood drained from my face to my toes, and I ran home to write this book.

Everyone is born with visual harmony. You have an instinctive feel for what looks good. You already know that you like certain color combinations better than others. You already know that something is wrong with the wallpaper in the bathroom. You already know what color looks best on you because your hand reaches first for the garments that have it. What you don't know is why you like certain colors and combinations of colors more than others. What you don't know is how to fine tune your innate color skills so that you can dress yourself and make purchasing decisions with complete confidence and accuracy.

The Blue Base/Yellow Base Color System will give you answers and techniques so that you can surround yourself with visual harmony—knowing what you're doing, understanding why you're doing it, and feeling the peace that such beauty creates.

The above photo shows typical Yellow Base colors. Similar Blue Base colors are used in the photo on the right. As you can see, some hue or tint of every color is in each color Spectrum.

The Blue Base/Yellow Base Color System

The year was 1928. An artist named Robert Dorr was working in Chicago making theatrical posters when he discovered that all colors—red, yellow, blue, black, white—and all the thousands of shades of these colors contained undertones of either blue or yellow. He found that all colors having blue pigmentation worked together in harmony, and all colors having yellow pigmentation worked together in harmony. Only when blue pigmented colors were mixed with yellow pigmented colors was there discord.

Becoming more and more fascinated with color harmony and how consistently people responded to it, Dorr observed that people, like colors, have a dominant blue (Spectrum 1) or yellow (Spectrum 2) pigmentation in their skin, eyes, and hair. The skin of Spectrum 1 people was rose-brown, rose-pink, or sallow-yellow. The skin of Spectrum 2 people was umber-brown, peach-pink, or golden-yellow.

When Dorr moved to the West Coast, he validated his findings through tests (using a spectrophotometer) on hundreds of thousands of men and women of all races and ages. He scientifically confirmed that people with Spectrum 1 coloring consistently purchased primarily Spectrum 1 colored merchandise, while people with Spectrum 2 coloring regularly bought Spectrum 2 colored merchandise. If a store typed its customers and kept records as to its customers' preferences, he wondered, wouldn't buyers then know more precisely how to select and balance inventory? Indeed they would! His findings impacted the marketplace dramatically.

When I inherited Robert Dorr's materials after his death in 1979, I continued his research through comprehensive studies conducted at Renae Knapp Color Institute Salons. We have found that when stores display goods whose colors harmonized within Blue Base or Yellow Base colors, sales go up. When goods are introduced that mix the two Spectrums, sales go down. People do not respond when the Spectrums are mixed because it is not pleasing to their eyes. Mixed Spectrum merchandise lands on the sale racks and in bargain basements.

What an aid to designers, manufacturers, and retailers understanding the Blue Base/Yellow Base Color System is. It lets them create goods in harmony! What a boon to consumers learning one's color group and buying within it is! This is invaluable information for a mother trying to help her son or daughter who is not in her color group buy school clothes. Husbands can now find the perfect birthday gift for their wives.

Our gift from Bob Dorr is the knowledge that every color we crave—whether to wear or to place in our environment—falls within Spectrum 1 colors or Spectrum 2 colors. It's simply a matter of pigments and blending them properly. Blue

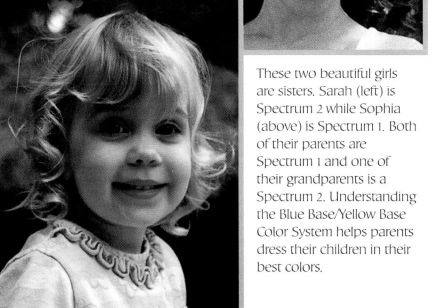

These two beautiful girls are sisters. Sarah (left) is Spectrum 2 while Sophia (above) is Spectrum 1. Both of their parents are Spectrum 1 and one of their grandparents is a Spectrum 2. Understanding the Blue Base/Yellow Base Color System helps parents dress their children in their best colors.

pigmented colors work with other blue pigmented colors; yellow pigmented colors work with other yellow pigmented colors. So long as we stay within one color Spectrum, we'll create harmony. If we mix the color groups, we create discord. The discord can be anywhere from shocking and obvious to subtle and "not too bad." But why settle for "not too bad," when "dynamite" and "smashing" are so easy to achieve?

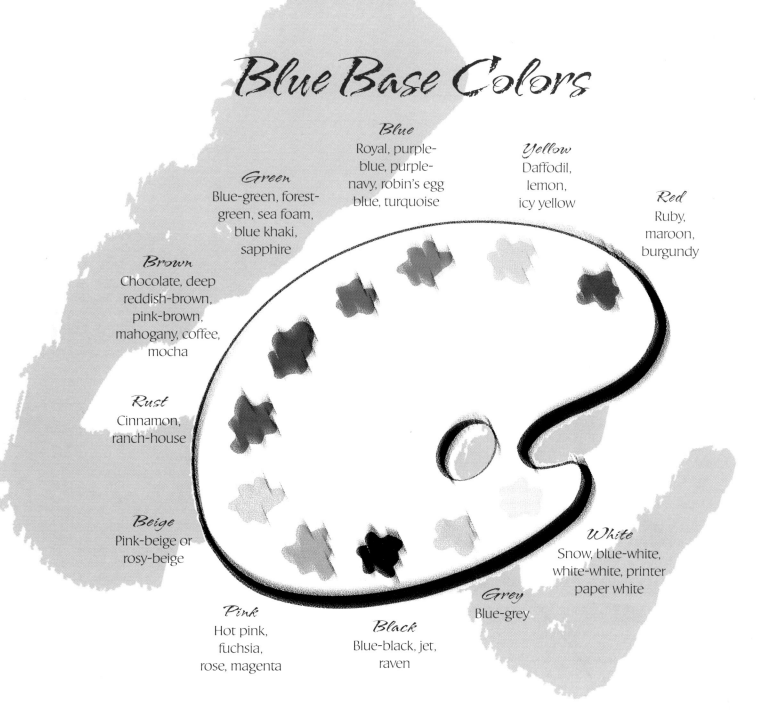

Blue Base Colors

Blue
Royal, purple-blue, purple-navy, robin's egg blue, turquoise

Yellow
Daffodil, lemon, icy yellow

Red
Ruby, maroon, burgundy

Green
Blue-green, forest-green, sea foam, blue khaki, sapphire

Brown
Chocolate, deep reddish-brown, pink-brown, mahogany, coffee, mocha

Rust
Cinnamon, ranch-house

White
Snow, blue-white, white-white, printer paper white

Beige
Pink-beige or rosy-beige

Grey
Blue-grey

Pink
Hot pink, fuchsia, rose, magenta

Black
Blue-black, jet, raven

Yellow Base Colors

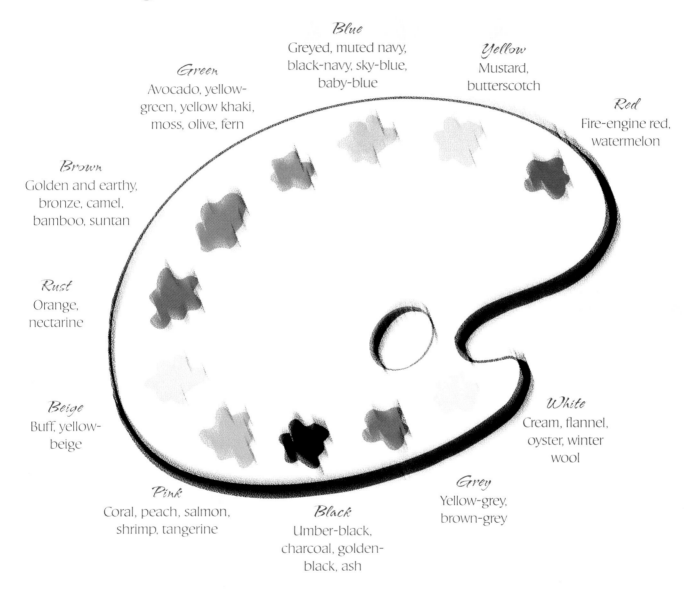

Blue
Greyed, muted navy, black-navy, sky-blue, baby-blue

Yellow
Mustard, butterscotch

Green
Avocado, yellow-green, yellow khaki, moss, olive, fern

Red
Fire-engine red, watermelon

Brown
Golden and earthy, bronze, camel, bamboo, suntan

Rust
Orange, nectarine

Beige
Buff, yellow-beige

White
Cream, flannel, oyster, winter wool

Pink
Coral, peach, salmon, shrimp, tangerine

Grey
Yellow-grey, brown-grey

Black
Umber-black, charcoal, golden-black, ash

Study the examples of colors for Blue Base/Yellow Base Colors, and you will get a feel for each in its proper classification. After studying the table, you will be well on the way to understanding why your expensive, rich looking blue-grey suit did not look particularly rich or wonderful with that ivory shirt you tried to wear with it. Go to your closet and test a different shirt—perhaps a blue-white or a rose-pink. Notice the miraculous change in the appearance of the suit. It will suddenly become expensive looking again, and you will feel excited about wearing it.

Every Color Has A Blue Base Or A Yellow Base

You will notice from the chart that there are no neutral colors. Black is not just black, and white is not just white. In other words, there is no such thing as a "universal" colored blouse, or a shirt that "goes with everything." Phrases such as "true blue" or "clear red" mean nothing. Only by working with pigments and ignoring labels can accuracy be achieved.

Blue Base/Yellow Base is not a "warm or cool" system. Each color group contains reds, blues, greens, browns, yellows, greys, blacks, and whites that relate warm, cool, greyed, and muted shades. You can assemble a wardrobe or a room décor that is neutral (soft, with only hints of color), or one that is vibrant (with bright color combinations), without ever going out of your preferred color group. You can put together outfits that are conservative and elegant, or outfits that are "way out" and alive with pizzazz—and you'll never lose color harmony.

The Blue Base black to the right looks clean and crisp with the Blue Base white. In contrast, the Yellow Base white looks dingy and dirty next to the Blue Base black above.

It is virtually impossible for you to make a mistake in combining colors when selecting from one Spectrum only. The Blue Base/Yellow Base Color System eliminates all trial and error and all guesswork and gives you a foolproof formula for success in working with color in all areas of your life. Blue Base/Yellow Base is not a fad or gimmick—it does not change with fashion trends. It's basic, unchanging, and as natural as you are.

Which Color Group Attracts You

Before you move on to the next chapter—where you will closely analyze your own coloring to determine which Spectrum you are—study the color palettes on pages four and five. Which palette attracts you immediately? Look objectively at each color palette—be sure to look at the whole palette and not at individual colors within it. You may like certain colors in both palettes. You may hate certain colors in both palettes. You may be an artist who just loves all color. Your entire home may be decorated in Yellow Base colors, yet you fit in better with Blue Base colors. None of this is important right now. Erase all preconceived notions—all your culturally conditioned responses—and simply ask yourself, "At my gut level, which color palette do I prefer overall?" The one you choose will help determine your colors for the rest of your life.

You will notice that every color except orange and magenta appears in each palette. Because of the heavy amount of yellow in orange, it is only in the Spectrum 2 color palette; because of the heavy amount of blue in magenta, it is only in the Spectrum 1 color palette. Nine times out of ten, people migrate to their color group—the same group that harmonizes with their skin, eyes, and hair. Nature does not mix pigments. It's a law of nature and harmony that colors flow harmoniously. Isn't it logical, then, that people would do the same? Trust yourself and your instincts. You are born into a color group, and you love the colors of you.

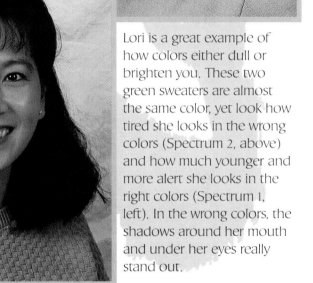

Lori is a great example of how colors either dull or brighten you. These two green sweaters are almost the same color, yet look how tired she looks in the wrong colors (Spectrum 2, above) and how much younger and more alert she looks in the right colors (Spectrum 1, left). In the wrong colors, the shadows around her mouth and under her eyes really stand out.

The Science Of Perfect Color

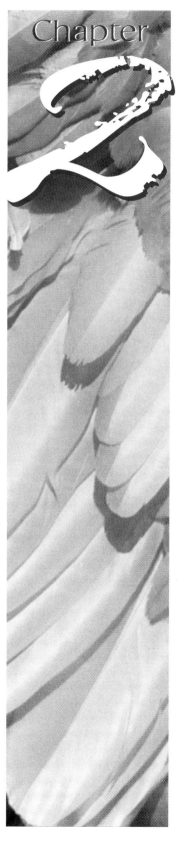

In the previous chapter, you chose the color group you felt you preferred. As we said earlier, the scientific findings are great that you have now discovered your correct color group. But just in case you're not sure, there are several ways of testing your choice.

You can very often know what group you fit into by paying attention to how you feel when you see things that don't seem to make you look as attractive as you like to look—such as the wrong make-up, eyeglasses, or hair color. You simply know something's not quite right. You may feel you need professional help or you think you just don't have what it takes. But remember, you do have what it takes—you are born with a built-in feeling for harmony.

The colors of most things we see are composed of primary pigments—red, yellow, blue, black, and white. All people worldwide—male and female, young and old, black, white, red, yellow, and brown—have individual skin, eye, and hair color. Personal coloring is a compilation of all the colors found in an individual's skin, eyes, and hair.

Analyzing What Nature Gave You

In attempting to analyze your coloring, keep a few important things in mind. First, we are talking about what nature gave you—not about what you do to yourself.

- Don't analyze hair that has been color treated, sun bleached, or exposed to a great deal of chlorine.

- Don't analyze skin that is laden with makeup.

- Don't analyze teeth that have been exposed to years of tobacco smoke, heavy tea, or coffee drinking.

- Don't analyze colors under artificial lights as they affect your coloring dramatically.

- Some antibiotics will discolor teeth in the formative years. If you have an illness for which you are taking heavy medication, it can alter your skin color. If you're a health food fan who eats lots and lots of carrots, be aware that the orange tints in your palms are caused by carotene, and are not your true coloring. Keep these in mind and don't analyze these areas.

All of these factors need to be taken into consideration when determining your personal color. Don't waste time proving you are the missing link—the first mixed-spectrum person on the face of the earth. Trust all the years of research, validation, and scientific backing that have gone into the Blue Base/Yellow Base Color System. It is 100% certain that your natural coloring is harmonious—you do not clash with yourself. In other words, if it is obvious that your hair is blue-grey, then it is obvious that you are a Spectrum 1 (Blue Base) person, and that's that! If it is obvious that there is orange around the irises of your eyes, you are a Spectrum 2 (Yellow Base) person, and that's that!

Trust the fact that you will always be in your color Spectrum. Your hair will turn grey in your Spectrum. Your moles and freckles will be in your Spectrum. You will tan in your Spectrum. But, most important, you will love your Spectrum, feel good in your Spectrum, and look harmonious in your Spectrum.

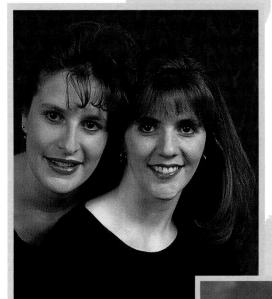

Katherine and Andrea (above) have very similar coloring. However, Katherine is Blue Base while Andrea is Yellow Base. The women on the right are another example that the tone of your skin does not determine your Spectrum. The model on the left is Yellow Base while the model on the right is Blue Base.

Lightness Or Darkness Does Not Affect Your Spectrum

The lightness and darkness of the skin has no bearing on what Spectrum you are. This might confuse you. You can be a very light skinned and fair Yellow Base person. You may say, "Well, I must be a Blue Base person, I'm so light." Not necessarily true! Or you may be a very dark brown-skinned Yellow Base person and think, "Well, I'm so dark, I must be a Blue Base person." Not necessarily true!

Because the jugular vein is in the neck, the blood runs closest to the surface of the skin there, so the neck is a good place to check out skin coloring. The eyes are also good to examine when attempting to determine your personal coloring. (Backs of wrists, so often used when testing makeup products, are totally inaccurate checkpoints.)

Here's a tip you may find useful: Blue Base people seem to show more facial hair than Yellow Base people. Blue Base men look as though they have a "five o'clock shadow," and Blue Base women seem to often have a "dirty" upper lip-line or mustache when wearing the opposite Spectrum—with a Yellow Base woman it's much more subtle.

A test I sometimes use in color typing is to place a person's hand on a peach fabric and then on a burgundy or deep raspberry fabric. The hand will appear to age, or to look older on the fabric that is in its opposite color group. With (Spectrum 1) olive skin, for example, the hand will seem greener and older when placed on the peach fabric than when placed on the burgundy fabric. This works for men and women of all ages and races.

The White Test

Another test I find helpful, especially in determining a man's Spectrum, is what I call the "White Test." Take a piece of very white Blue Base fabric, and a piece of off-white (not beige) Yellow Base fabric. Drape these under his chin and you can easily see which one makes him look too yellow, too beardy, too pale, or just not

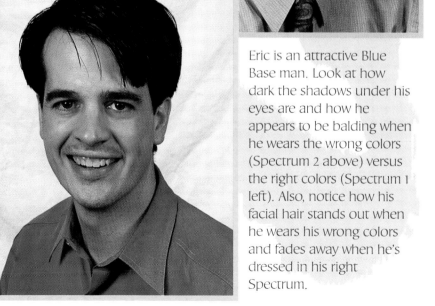

Eric is an attractive Blue Base man. Look at how dark the shadows under his eyes are and how he appears to be balding when he wears the wrong colors (Spectrum 2 above) versus the right colors (Spectrum 1 left). Also, notice how his facial hair stands out when he wears his wrong colors and fades away when he's dressed in his right Spectrum.

as sharp as the other. The Blue Base white will make the teeth of a Yellow Base person seem too yellow. The Yellow Base white will look a little dirty (ring around the collar) next to the whites of a Blue Base person's eyes, teeth, and hair (especially if the hair is starting to grey). In both cases, the natural color harmony will be lost.

As you analyze and study yourself objectively, it will become apparent to you that colors selected from your color group flatter you most. You will look and feel exciting in them. Colors in your opposite color group will do little for you—at best, you'll look uninteresting and boring. You will see this even with something as basic as navy blue. Spectrum 1 navy is a purple type navy and looks exciting and rich on a Blue Base person. Yellow Base navy will look "okay" on a Blue Base person, but why settle for okay? On a Yellow Base person, Blue Base navy looks too harsh, a little garish and overpowering. We see a garment wearing a person rather than a person wearing a garment when they're dressed in the wrong Spectrum. The Yellow Base person needs a more greyed, black navy.

Katherine is a great example of the difference the right colors can make. Look at how much more vibrant and natural she looks in her correct Blue Base colors (right) instead of her wrong Yellow Base colors (above).

You're going to spend money dressing yourself, whether at a discount house or at the finest boutique. Yet no matter where you choose to buy your clothes, and no matter how much or how little money you spend on them, the principle is the same—you will look more exciting and be the star of your outfit only when its colors are in your Spectrum.

Personal Coloring

The following charts are provided to help you see the differences between Spectrum 1 (Blue Base) and Spectrum 2 (Yellow Base) as they apply to skin tone, teeth, eye color, and hair color.

Skin Tone

Spectrum 1 (Blue Base)

Caucasian

Blue undertone produces a somewhat rose-pink complexion: hands will be pink, with perhaps purple or rose-pink knuckles.

African American, Black

Blue undertone produces a visible blue cast in very dark black skin, and a smoky or umber tone in lighter black skin.

Asian, Hispanic, Native American, Mediterranean

Blue undertone produces a reddish brown or smoky blue cast, yellow in skin will be sallow, with a green/grey cast.

Spectrum 2 (Yellow Base)

Caucasian

Prominent yellow undertones produce a peach-pink tone; hands will be yellow or golden with peach-pink knuckles.

African American, Black

Yellow undertone produces a definite gold tone to the skin.

Asian, Hispanic, Native American, Mediterranean

Yellow undertone produces a golden cast to the skin. Actual yellow in the skin will have a definite golden tone.

Tooth Color

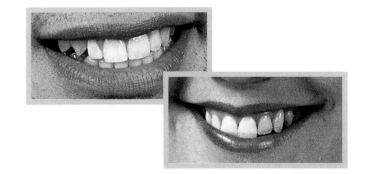

Spectrum 1 (Blue Base)

Blue-white, grey-white

Visible caps and fillings should be consistent and in harmony with your personal coloring.

Spectrum 2 (Yellow Base)

Creamy white

Visible caps and fillings should be consistent and in harmony with your personal coloring.

Eye Color

Yellow is very often found mixed with the various colors around the iris of hazel eyes—this can be a Spectrum 1 yellow or a Spectrum 2 gold.

Spectrum 1 (Blue Base)   Spectrum 2 (Yellow Base)

Deep brown, almost black eyes with the blue ring around the iris are typical Spectrum 1 eyes.

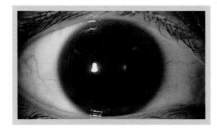

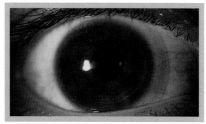

The flat-navy ring around this brown iris is a clear sign of a Spectrum 2 eye. Also, notice how peach the skin around the eye is.

Blue Base people can have brilliant blue eyes, These will tend to have a blue-grey cast to them.

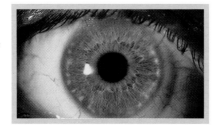

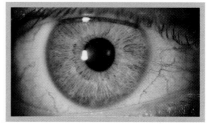

This is a common Spectrum 2 eye color. Notice how this eye is more grey-blue than the Blue Based, blue-grey eye to the far left. Also the very orange veins in this eye signal a Spectrum 2 person.

This is a very common Blue Base eye color. Notice the reddish-brown specks, and the lemon yellow coloring.

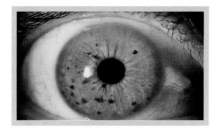

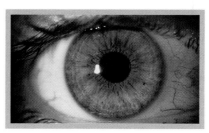

With Spectrum 2 hazel eyes, the yellow is very golden.

This is a typical reddish-brown eye color. Also notice the very pink skin around the eyes and the purple-blue ring around the iris.

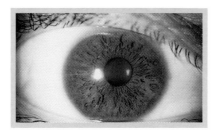

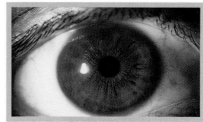

Compare this eye with the one to the left. The Spectrum 2 eye is much more orange-brown while the Spectrum 1 eye to the far left is more reddish-brown.

Hair Color

If hair has been treated with chemicals (including all rinses or coloring agents), do not use it as an indicator of your Spectrum, unless you use only natural grow-out.

Spectrum 1 (Blue Base)

Blonde

Platinum, ash, smoky undertone, lemon yellow (not gold) highlights

Red

Cinnamon, auburn, reddish brown

Brown

Pink cast to the brown color, (The color is often referred to as "mousy," usually people with this will highlight their hair.) dark chestnut

Black

Jet, blue-black (Spectrum 1 black people have a shiny finish to their hair.)

White

Blue-grey, snowy white, smoky blue, purple highlights, silver

Spectrum 2 (Yellow Base)

Blonde

Golden, honey, strawberry

Red

Orange rust, golden carrot

Brown

Golden brown

Black

Off-black, almost brown (Yellow Base black people have a matte—not so shiny—finish to their hair.)

White

Cream-white, overall pale yellow tone

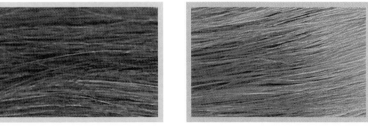

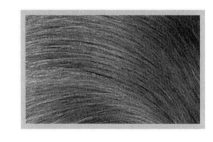

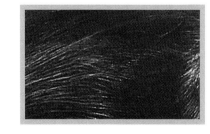

In Blue Base hair color, red highlights are often present, even if red is not the predominant color. This will be an auburn red, not orange red. Men will have these auburn red hairs in their mustache or beard.

In Yellow Base hair color, golden highlights and orange red highlights are common. Do not confuse these with the auburn red highlights of Blue Base hair color. Men will have orange red and golden red hairs in their mustache or beard.

Maximize Haircolor, Eyewear, And Cosmetics

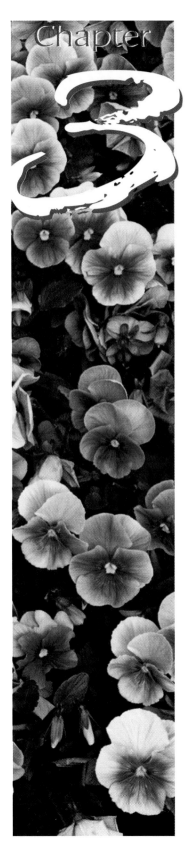

Even though you are now looking at color in a way you've never looked at color before (and are probably excited to buy your next eye shadow, business suit, or living room carpet!), there's something very important you must do first. You need to analyze your light source and to be aware of light and how it affects the colors you see. There may be colors in your skin, eyes, and hair, or in the clothing, eye shadow, or décor you select, that you won't be able to see in the current light.

Check Your Light Source

All color is seen through light. There is no color without light. Light comes from various sources: the sun, incandescent and fluorescent bulbs, mercury vapor lamps, candles, and so forth. Color results from the interactions of the light source, the object on which the light is focused, and the physiological functioning of the tiny rods and cones in our eyes (if the latter are not 100% functional, we're color blind to a degree).

There are also psychological factors that affect our perception of color: if mean Miss Grundy, your second-grade teacher, often wore a certain color, you may go through life disliking it. If your favorite granny wore a certain color frequently, you may always favor it. A combination of physiological and psychological factors determines how we see color.

Isaac Newton

In 1666, when Isaac Newton flashed a beam of seemingly colorless sunlight through a prism to reveal a red-orange-yellow-green-blue-purple-violet ribbon of color with gradations in between, he showed us that the sunbeam wasn't colorless at all, but filled with color. However, because of the various light sources affecting our daily perceptions of color, we rarely see the full Spectrum. Often we see distortions of the true color. Some common fluorescent tubes may reflect back to us only blue and green, and others may reflect back only yellow. Candles, for example, produce light at the red-yellow end of the Spectrum, revealing no blue, purple, or violet. Ever had dinner by candlelight when the table was set with a navy blue tablecloth or dark blue china? The cloth or china will look black. Personal coloring should be determined in the daylight if at all possible. True color, according to the experts, is most evident at 11:00 AM on a clear day.

Now that you have determined your preferred Spectrum, you need to do some fine-tuning within it. Even though everyone looks best in either Blue Base or Yellow Base colors, people are still unique in how the colors from their Spectrum look on them.

Although you will always look harmonious if you wear any of the colors in your Spectrum, by focusing in on those colors found specifically in your personal coloring (your skin, eyes, and hair) you will create an appearance that is exciting, and has individuality and style. You will look alive, healthy, and will radiate a special glow. People will comment on how terrific you look, not just on how terrific-looking your outfit is.

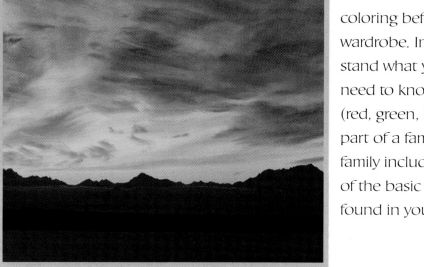

Light allows us to see the colors that surround us. However, the colors we see can appear to be different hues or tints in different lights.

Think through your personal coloring before you rethink your wardrobe. In order to clearly understand what you are looking for, you need to know that each basic color (red, green, blue, yellow, et cetera) is part of a family of colors. The color family includes tones, tints, and shades of the basic color, all of which may be found in your skin, eyes, and hair.

Skin

As you look for the many colors in your skin, look carefully to see if you have plum (Spectrum 1) or purple (Spectrum 2) undertones in your skin. The plums or purples can be found in the skin along the upper side of the nose, under the eye areas, or sometimes in the lips. The cheek area will very often have a strong amount of plum or purple as well.

If you have determined that you are a Spectrum 1 person, but you have not found plum (your skin is strongly rose pink instead), then the plum and lavender color groups are not as exciting on you as pinks, raspberries, and very rosy burgundies.

If you are a Spectrum 2 person and find only pink (not as much brown and peach) in your skin, then oranges and strong peach colors will not look as attractive on you as shrimp and salmon. If you are a Spectrum 2 person with more brown and peach in your skin, pinks will not be as striking on you as the peach colors, including peachy browns and rusts.

An exception to wearing colors from your personal coloring can be found in the color yellow, which is only good to wear if it can be found in your eyes. Do not wear yellow if it is present in your skin. If you're olive-skinned or Asian, leave yellow garments alone.

African Americans, or other dark-skinned people, will have the same colors present in their skin, and should use the same approach. Remember, the darkness or lightness of one's skin has no bearing on the individual's Spectrum or personal colors. Spectrum 1 black skin contains plums, rose-pinks, and burgundies. This means that they will look fantastic in rosy browns, burgundies, and blue-pinks.

Spectrum 2 African skin will have more yellow-brown present, and even orange-rusts and shrimp or peach colors. Brown is obviously

Thomas, a handsome Spectrum 1 person, looks classy and his skin tones look rich in his Blue Base colors (left). In the wrong colors, (Spectrum 2 above) Thomas looks sallow and ashen.

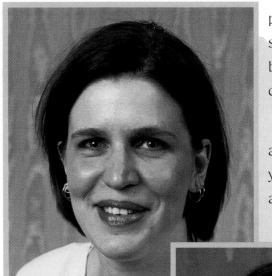

present in the skin of Africans, and therefore, they will look striking in brown so long as it is a brown in their Spectrum. Spectrum 1 black people look best in chocolate and reddish browns, and Spectrum 2 black people look dynamite in golden, earthy browns.

It's important to study your skin colors very specifically, not just generally. You will then be able to zero in on the color families that dominate your personal coloring. If you have a hard time seeing yourself objectively, ask a good friend to help you.

Cynthia is a great example of how colors found in your eyes are accentuated when you surround yourself with the same colors. When you look at the top picture, you can see how none of Cynthia's features stand out when she wears her wrong Spectrum 2 colors. In the bottom picture, Cynthia is in her correct Spectrum 1 colors and she looks much more balanced and natural. The middle picture shows Cynthia surrounded by the same color found in her eyes. Notice how her eyes appear so much more brilliant when she is surrounded by those colors.

Eyes

Eyes are never just one solid color. They are a combination of several colors giving the impression of one color. Stretch your vision to see all the nuances of eye color. Get a large magnifying mirror if that will help.

To find the colors in your eyes, take a super close look at the colored part—the iris. Do you see brown feathering into green? The exact tones, tints, and shades of brown in your eyes are you, and will look great translated into clothing. The greens you see are your greens to wear. In Spectrum 1 people, these may be soft blue-greens with a lot of grey, or possibly some lime greens, or even dark forest greens. Check also for blue-khaki. In Spectrum 2 people, these may be deep olive, moss, or avocado-type greens. Check also for yellow khaki.

Can you see some yellow in the iris? You will look terrific in yellow if it is present in your eyes. Check carefully. Yellow is a difficult color for most people to wear. It must be found in the eyes, not the skin, if it is to wear well.

If you have blue eyes, do you see a lot of white in the blue? If so, white will be even more striking on you (especially if you have white-grey hair to match). Check the blue. Is it the bright Spectrum 1 royal blue, or the more muted Spectrum 1 blue-grey? If green is present in the blue, aqua blue-greens—the colors of the Mediterranean sea—will be great for you. Sky blue eyes signal Spectrum 2, and most Spectrum 2 blues and navies are perfect color choices for people with Spectrum 2 blue eyes.

If you have brown eyes—chocolate brown (Spectrum 1) or golden brown (Spectrum 2)—a plum (Spectrum 1) or purple (Spectrum 2) ring around the iris is usually present. Depending on which color is present in your brown eyes, Spectrum 1 plum or Spectrum 2 purple is a dynamite color for you to wear.

Navy is found around the iris of almost all eyes, thus making navy (Spectrum 1 purple-navy or Spectrum 2 black or grey-navy) an excellent color choice for most individuals, whether they have blue, brown, or hazel eyes.

Do It With Color

By now, you have probably thought of certain colors that are uniquely you. Perhaps you have noticed a strong amount of black in your hair coloring and around the irises of your eyes. You may also have noticed that you have a lot of raspberry, burgundy, and pink in your skin. You may see deep blue-greens in your eyes between the iris and the pupil. You can see that your coloring is made up of distinct tones, tints, and shades of several color families.

Now choose the family of colors that you love the most and feel the most exciting in, choose all the colors from that color family (not

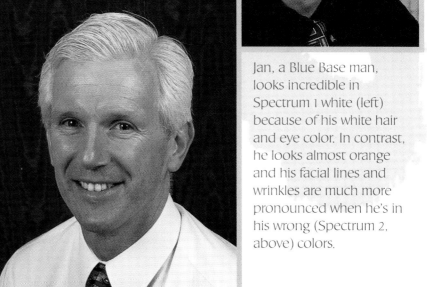

Jan, a Blue Base man, looks incredible in Spectrum 1 white (left) because of his white hair and eye color. In contrast, he looks almost orange and his facial lines and wrinkles are much more pronounced when he's in his wrong (Spectrum 2, above) colors.

one specific tone, tint, or shade), and make that collection of colors your pivotal colors. Your pivotal colors are anchor points in your closet—the colors around which your clothing selection revolves.

When you have determined your pivotal colors from a close examination of your personal coloring, use these colors the most; make these the ones you always come back to. These colors give you stability and flow. Carry them in your closet during both summer and winter. Have tones, tints, and shades of the pivotal colors, as well as supporting accessories. If you have only one handbag, go pivotal. If you have only one raincoat, go pivotal. This is the hub of your personal colors, and the rest of your closet's contents should radiate harmoniously from this collection of colors.

If you have a limited wardrobe or have no need for a lot of clothes in your particular job or lifestyle, simply stick to your pivotal colors. If you want to develop a larger wardrobe, add colors from your second and third color families to your closet. The particular pieces you choose should be geared to your lifestyle and particular needs. There are two classes that we teach at Renae Knapp Color Institute Salons that offer invaluable information about your personal colors: Color Dynamics and Dressing Distinctively. Check Appendix C for more information on those classes.

Luminosity

Luminosity, here, means the brightness or dullness of color. It does not mean light versus dark, as in tones, tints, and shades. There are light pastel colors that are just as vibrant as some dark colors. The rule with regard to the luminosity of a color is simple: never overpower your own natural coloring. The luminosity level or brightness of the color you are wearing, using in cosmetics, coloring your hair with, or choosing for your eyewear, should enhance your features but not override them.

By analyzing your individual coloring and selecting the colors that

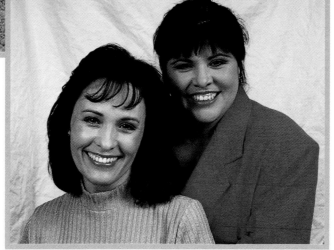

Juanita and Maria, both Blue Base Hispanic women, are a perfect example of high and low luminosity. Juanita (far right) looks striking in the hot pink jacket she's wearing. If Maria (right) wore the hot pink, she would look overpowered even though it is in her correct Spectrum. The broken blush samples above are another example of high and low luminosity Spectrum 1 colors.

complement it, both with the correct color and luminosity level, you have enhanced what nature gave you, and are ready to put a confident foot forward.

Cosmetics

No cosmetic or hair color product can enhance your natural beauty if you select a color not in your color group. You may look more painted, but you won't look more attractive. Only by selecting cosmetic and hair colors that harmonize with your natural coloring can you achieve a look that brings your eyes forward, evens out your skin tones, and projects an alert-looking, healthy, and natural glow.

First, let's deal with cosmetic colors. There are hundreds of shades of lipstick, nail polish, and blushers. They can be dark, light, muted, or frosted. Yet every one of these shades derives from six basic reds—three are Spectrum 1 colors, and three are Spectrum 2 colors.

Spectrum 1 Colors	Spectrum 2 Colors
Mulberry red	Rust red
Blue red	Orange red
Magenta red	Vermilion red

Eye shadows, pencils, and foundations also come in a wide range of color, tints, and shades. These, too, should be selected from your color group.

The amount of frosting added to a cosmetic color increases its level of luminosity but does not change its basic color. Cosmetics are classified as matte, low pearl, medium pearl, and high pearl. Whichever your color group, it is important not to overpower your own natural coloring with make-up that

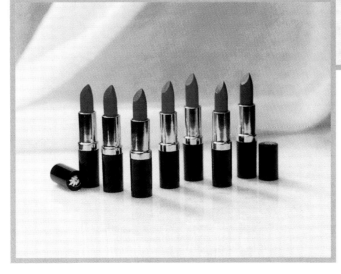

Lipstick is one of the most visible facial colors. It is critical that you use the right Spectrum and luminosity of lipstick for your face. Choose a blush that corresponds with your lipstick.

is too intense. If your eyes are a muted green or brown, then eye shadow should be low-luminosity—matte or low pearl, but never high pearl. If your skin pigmentation is of a high luminosity, then the most flattering color would probably be one that is medium or high pearl.

The older we get, the more careful we must be in working with frosting and luminosity level in our make-up. Our skin may lose some of its color strength, so make-up should become softer, not brighter.

Avoiding Mixed Spectrum Make-Up

A well-known make-up artist once said that one of the things that disturbed him the most was women who wore make-up colors that clashed with their clothes. As an example, he described a woman who dressed in a rust-colored blouse and wore a raspberry blusher. To avoid such a situation, he suggested buying clothes that dramatize the eyes and set off the hair and then using make-up that complements the natural features. Without actually using the words Blue Base/Yellow Base, he was really talking about not mixing Spectrum 1 and Spectrum 2 colors.

Never mix Spectrum 1 and Spectrum 2 colors on the same facial palette. Your growing understanding of the Blue Base/Yellow Base Color System will help you avoid this common mistake. Instead, you'll learn to create a totally coordinated cosmetics case to accompany a totally coordinated you.

Sound simple? It really is, once you understand and have a basic knowledge of color and how it works. Blue Base and Yellow Base colors just don't mix. But, when you're purchasing cosmetics, how do you know which items have a Blue Base and which have a Yellow Base?

Because of increased awareness of the importance of color, there are cosmetologists and

Color harmony or discord is never more apparent than with make-up. Because make-up is layered, mixing Yellow Base and Blue Base colors makes individual colors stand out instead of blending naturally together. Mixing Spectrums makes you look painted while harmonizing same Spectrum colors makes you look natural.

aestheticians who know about Blue Base and Yellow Base make-up. I also have a team of associates around the world at Renae Knapp Color Institute Salons who can help you find your absolute best make-up colors. Call my office and tell them which color base you require. Someone will connect you with a local Renae Knapp Color Institute Salon Associate who can show you cosmetics that fit your Spectrum.

Renae Knapp Body Care and Renae Knapp Cosmetic products are the only products in the world founded on the science of the Blue Base/Yellow Base Color System. You will find your very best colors and not waste time on something inappropriate and potentially wrong for your coloring if you use Renae Knapp products. The problem with mixed Spectrum make-up is compounded because it's difficult to see true color value in the lighting at a department store cosmetics counter. This is why I've taken the guesswork out of buying cosmetics and instead I'm saving you time and money while helping you achieve your very best look.

There are too many techniques and pointers that simplify cosmetic application to list here. Study Appendix A or visit a Renae Knapp Color Institute Salon for personal assistance to learn more about simplifying and perfecting the daily process of make-up application.

Remember, when you wear cosmetics in your opposite Spectrum, lines and wrinkles become much more pronounced. You will look tired, under the weather, or actually ill. You will lose much of your attractiveness and credibility. Cosmetics are worn near and around our most important personal coloring aspects— jugular vein, lips, iris, cheeks, eyelids, and hair. If you choose the wrong Spectrum, you place yourself at a tremendous disadvantage when meeting new people or going to an important event where you must sell yourself.

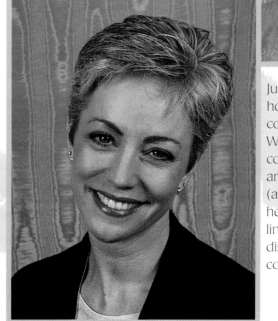

Julie is a great example of how important wearing the correct make-up color is. When she wears her wrong colors she appears tired and her skin looks uneven (above). Her skin becomes healthy and balanced the lines and wrinkles almost disappear in her correct colors (left).

Eyewear

Your eyes are your most important feature, the one that everyone relates to, the one from which your expressions and personality shine forth. If you wear contact lenses or glasses, it's crucial that they complement your natural coloring, style, and "put-together" look. People should look at you and say, "What an attractive person; look at those wonderful eyes," not "Oh, glasses."

For many years it was considered such a miracle that science and technology could help people see better with eyeglasses that few people complained about the limited choice of frames. Indeed, great grandma and great grandpa had only one choice—a small, round wire frame. Few looked attractive in these frames and many people looked ridiculous. Next came a plain gold unisex frame that also looked ridiculous.

Today we have unlimited choices of shape, color, style, and workmanship. Glasses are now perceived by most people as attractive accessories, not just functional adjuncts to vision. While the eyewear fashion phenomenon skyrocketed, the optical profession made great strides in acquiring the expertise to help consumers with color selection on a sophisticated level.

Many optical professionals are now trained in the Blue Base/Yellow Base Color System. In fact, Vision Industry Council of America (the industry association for optical professionals) uses the Blue Base/Yellow Base Color System and related materials exclusively. You can call VICA (see Appendix F) for information regarding an optical store near you that uses the Blue Base/Yellow Base Color System.

You need to be aware of what to look for when selecting your eyewear. Your knowledge of the Blue Base/Yellow Base Color System and the following rules will help you avoid costly mistakes:

• Never buy lenses that mix Blue Base and Yellow Base colors, or lenses tinted in the Spec-

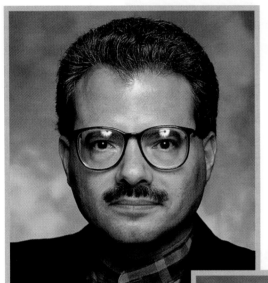

Glasses should compliment your facial features, not over power them. In the photo above, the frames are too large. The frames in the picture to the right compliment and show off the facial features.

trum opposite yours. To enhance the coloring of your skin, hair, and eyes, only select eyewear in the colors in your personal color group.

- Never buy a tint so dark that it obscures your eye area (except for sunglasses). The frame and lens tint of your sunglasses should also be in your color group.

- Always note the color placement on the frame, and be sure it helps achieve balance and proportion given the shape of your face.

The color of your lenses is as important to your overall appearance as frame selection. Untinted lenses distort the eyes slightly, either accenting bags or circles under them or making the eyes look dull and old. When done artistically and in your color Spectrum, tinting softens the eye area, enhances natural coloring, and helps your eyes come forward from behind the lenses. When done poorly, tinting detracts from your eyes' appearance.

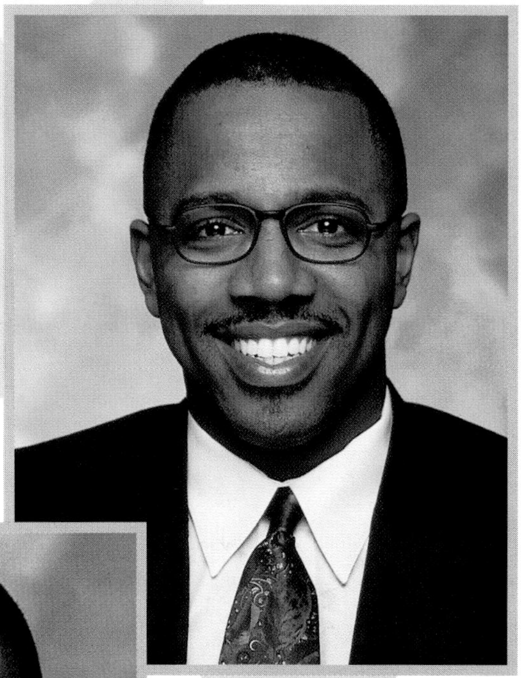

Lens Tinting

Lens tinting should be an art. Unfortunately, many of its practitioners have not been trained to assess skin tones to help you select the proper tint. The professional with no knowledge of color may tint your lenses in the Spectrum opposite yours. All of us have noticed these disasters—people wearing lenses that make their eyes look sick or people who look as though someone took a marker and drew a ring around their eyes. When the tint clashes with a person's natural coloring, the focal point of the face becomes the two round circles over the eyes.

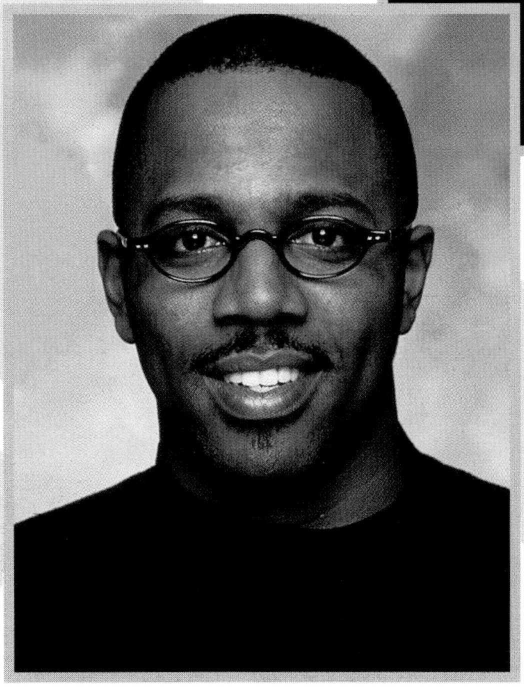

Tints should be subtle. They should enhance, not obscure, the individual's own natural features. If a person is Blue Base, the tint in the lower lens area should pick up the rose-pink of the skin tones. If a person is Yellow Base, the lower lens tint should pick up the peach-pink

The shape and size of frames should accent good points on the face. In the picture above, the large square frames draw attention to themselves while the frames in the picture to the left draw attention to the whole face.

skin tones, blending the skin and lens harmoniously. There should never be a dramatic separation of tints, skin tones, and frame. Tinting of the upper lens area should pick up skin tones, eye colors, or eye shadow colors (such as soft browns, blues, and greys). Lenses tinted in the wrong color for you will make you look as though you're bug-eyed or staring. Your eyes will look painted onto your face. Remember that contact lenses should be the correct tint, also.

Make-Up Under Those Frames

Very often, women who wear glasses tell me they don't need make-up because their glasses are tinted or their frames are very decorative and that does the job for them. Wrong! Women who wear glasses, tinted or untinted, decorative or not, need make-up more than other women. It helps give definition to the eye area. As light reflects off the lenses, the eyes get lost underneath. Thicker lenses enlarge the eye area, causing circles, wrinkles, and flaws to become more pronounced. With make-up, especially cover-up cream in the eye area, the eyes themselves (not the surrounding flaws) become the focal point and look more youthful. Apply the basic rules of eye make-up (see Appendix A), then use the following special pointers for eyeglass wearers, and notice the difference!

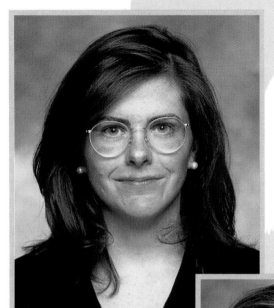

The photo above is a perfect example of how choosing the wrong frames and not wearing make-up are very uncomplimentary. The photo to the right clearly shows how much more professional and put together an individual can look with the right frames and make-up on.

Since glasses will emphasize the circles and lines under your eyes, it is important to wear a cover cream or powder to give a smoother look. Go with creams and powders, not sticks, for a softer, more natural look. Under glasses, the eyes of nearsighted people look smaller, so a light shade of eye shadow on the lids helps bring the eyes forward. Farsighted people should use a darker eye shadow on the eyelids, to avoid a "bug-eyed" look. Remember: light brings forward, dark diminishes. Eyeliner and lots of mascara help give definition to the eyes of nearsighted and farsighted people who wear glasses.

They also finish off your look. Tell your optical professional that you are a Blue Base or Yellow Base person and want eyewear that enhances your natural facial characteristics and features.

Hair Coloring

Hair color is essentially the one permanent or semipermanent cosmetic. This makes it critical that your hair be colored in your Spectrum. Since so many women highlight, frost, foil, tint, or color their hair at some point in their lives, it's important to think about the effect hair coloring has on your total look. Increasingly, men are also coloring their hair and the number of men wearing toupees and having donor hair transplants has risen sharply in recent years.

Since coloring hair is a chemical process to which people react individually, it is impossible for manufacturers to accurately label hair coloring products as to color Spectrum. Therefore, colors must be tested on the individual before a choice of product and color is made.

If you color your hair now or are contemplating doing so, make absolutely sure that the color you get is in your color group. This brings up the inherent problem with hair color and the professional hair colorist: most hair colorists will color a client's hair based on the colorist's own color preferences. In other words, a Spectrum 1 hair colorist will find it in much better "taste" to color everyone's hair in Blue Base colors. A Spectrum 2 hair colorist will find it in better taste to do everyone in Yellow Base colors. Why? Well, we are all programmed to see color through our own perceptions. We have an innate sense for what we believe is better and more attractive.

We gravitate to our own Spectrums because it feels good to us; it feels right. Here are some important points to remember when coloring your hair:

- If foiling or highlighting your hair blonde, remember: golden blonde for Yellow Base and ash blonde for Blue

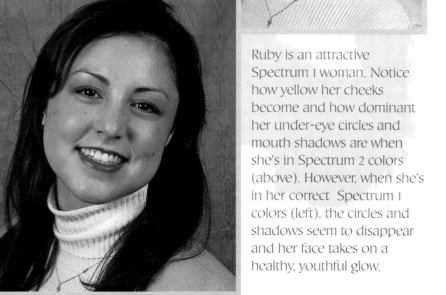

Ruby is an attractive Spectrum 1 woman. Notice how yellow her cheeks become and how dominant her under-eye circles and mouth shadows are when she's in Spectrum 2 colors (above). However, when she's in her correct Spectrum 1 colors (left), the circles and shadows seem to disappear and her face takes on a healthy, youthful glow.

Base. For your most credible and powerful look, highlights should come close to the same color of your hair when you were a child. If you are not sure that blonde is right for you, ask yourself if your hair turns some shade of blonde in strong sun—say, after two weeks in Maui? If you have light colored eyes or blonde flecks in your iris, match the blonde in the iris of your eye and you have a guaranteed winner.

- Never cover grey hair with the opposite Spectrum. If you do, your hair will look flat, dull, and artificial. Try to come close to the natural color, or slightly lighter if there is heavy grey.

- Avoid harsh chemical color treatments that cause brassy and artificial undertones to appear. The idea of hair color is to enhance and beautify, not to make it noticeable.

- If you are a Blue Base, avoid color processes that only lift the hair a few shades. More than likely your hair will turn to a Yellow Base and the look will be a "fake" one. Darker ash (Blue Base) blondes will more than likely require bleach to lift the hair out of Yellow Base.

If you are unsure that you are getting the expertise and color standard you prefer, call my office at 1-888-395-9323 for the nearest Renae Knapp Color Institute Salon location. We have many experienced and thoroughly trained hair colorists all over the world who can help you get it right the first time, and avoid the embarrassment of bad hair color.

Now that your make-up and hair color are appropriate for you, you are on your way to looking and feeling totally put together, totally harmonious, and totally beautiful.

Hair Coloring Guidelines

Hair	Spectrum 1 Colors
Black	Raven, jet, blue
Brown	Reddish, coffee, rose
Red	Cinnamon, auburn
Blonde	Platinum, pink
Grey	Silver, snowy, white blue

Hair Coloring Guidelines

Hair	Spectrum 2 Colors
Black	Charcoal-grey, ash
Brown	Golden, warm chestnut
Red	Bronze, carrot-orange
Blonde	Beige, champagne, honey golden
Grey	Warm, golden, creamy white

Incorrectly colored hair not only looks unfashionable, but sends a clear message that you are trying to change who you are. Correctly colored hair looks natural. These boxes list correct hair colors for each Spectrum. For an example of these colors, please refer to the chart on page 15.

The Do's And Don'ts Of Shopping

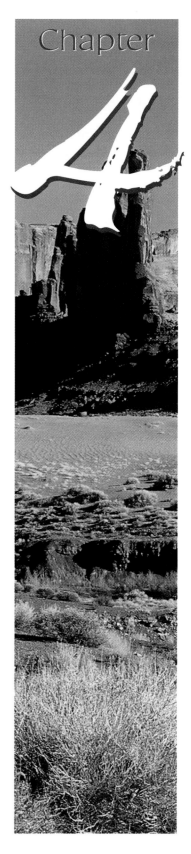

By learning what I teach in this chapter, you can save yourself a lot of money, and avoid the pitfalls and negative reactions associated with buying articles of your opposite Spectrum colors, or mixed Spectrum colors.

First, always purchase your best or pivotal colors—the colors that occur in your eyes, skin and hair. These colors are those from your personal coloring that are dynamic on you and make you come alive and look stunning. They are also colors that give you a psychological edge on life when you wear them. You just know you can do anything when you have these colors on. They are *must have* colors in your closet. You can't live without them.

Save Time And Money

> *"I have two objectives now: 1) To not waste time,*
> *2) To come to the truth as quickly as possible."*
>
> *Christopher Reeve*

The Blue Base/Yellow Base Color System is extremely beneficial for two reasons. First, you save a tremendous amount of time deciding what to wear. You have a working tool which helps you get ready each morning. Every item should be able to mix and match with other items. If it does, you will now have a full, working wardrobe. You will have a strong anchor point in your closet. You can add as much as you want and it will just flow into the system you have already created. Each item added will create several new outfits, not just one. Each purchase will be based on a science of putting you together. Secondly, you save great amounts of money by purchasing "sure winners" instead of "I'm having a bad day" items that end up at the back of your closet. So, let's get into how and where to buy for your own color Spectrum.

Demographics And Blue Base/Yellow Base

In the Pacific Northwest, where I lived most of my life, 85% of the population is Blue Base. Consequently, most people in Seattle, Portland, and Vancouver like and purchase Blue Base merchandise. However, 80% of the southwestern United States, where I currently live, is Yellow Base. It is difficult for a Blue Base person to find his or her best colors in San Diego or Phoenix. The northeastern United States is also predominantly Blue Base, while the Southeast is mostly Yellow Base. The Midwest is an even mix of both. In Japan, the population is 75% Blue Base and 25% Yellow Base. China and Hong Kong are 65% Yellow Base and 35% Blue Base.

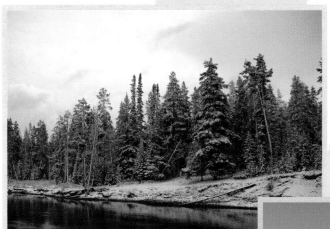

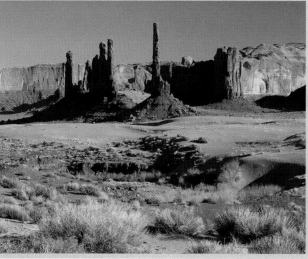

Depending on what area of the country you live in, you may have a difficult time finding goods to buy that are in your Spectrum. This is because portions of the United States are predominantly Blue Base or Yellow Base and thus attract more of those people.

With that said, depending where you live, you will have an easier or harder time finding things you like or that work for you. Because Nordstrom is based out of Seattle and the Nordstrom stores themselves are Blue Base, they will usually hire Blue Base people (remember: likes attract). Those Blue Base people will likely hire Blue Based buyers who will then purchase Blue Base clothing and accessories for the stores. That is a simplistic example, but generally a true one. You can usually tell the color base of the person who runs the store by the colors in the merchandise being sold there. We gravitate to what we are because we feel it is in better taste. Therefore, the store owner may feel he or she is doing you a favor by selling you merchandise in "good taste," rather than merchandise he or she feels is "tacky."

My son recently went to a major department store to buy a tie in the men's department. He is a Spectrum 1 and was very specific with the Spectrum 2 sales clerk as to the color of tie he wanted. The clerk was horrified and felt it his job to save my son from committing such a blunder. My son simply wanted a plain burgundy tie (Spectrum 1), and couldn't get the clerk to take it out of the display case. The clerk kept bringing out orange and golden colored (Spectrum 2) ties.

Due to my son's extensive knowledge of the Blue Base/Yellow Base Color System, he was not persuaded by the persistent clerk to get a different tie. After my son finally insisted on the burgundy tie, the clerk just walked away and let some other employee finalize the sale.

When you are armed with the Blue Base/Yellow Base Color System, you assume control of your purchasing decisions without following the habits and preferences of others. To make things easier, shop in stores offering *your* colors. This type of store will naturally feel good to you. If you need assistance, look for a salesperson that is also in your color Spectrum.

Lighting

As I previously mentioned, lighting is critical for color correctness. Light is the twin of color. Without light, there would be no color. Most stores have bad lighting, but direct sunlight is not that good, either. Direct sunlight can easily distort color. When you want to analyze something in the store, look for a simple light bulb—the kind that spotlight the mannequins. Otherwise, indirect sunlight is the best color indicator.

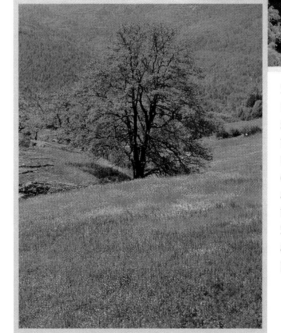

Since people naturally feel more comfortable when surrounded by colors from their Spectrum, and since they tend to believe that colors from their Spectrum are more appealing, regions that are predominantly one Spectrum or the other attract that Spectrum of people.

When in doubt, go with your first impression or "gut level" sense of a color. That will usually be the right one for you. An excellent tool to take with you shopping is the Renae Knapp "Personal Pro" Fan Deck. To order this pocket-size color dictionary, call us at 1-888-395-9323. We will send you a small color dictionary that will assist you in determining correct colors at the store. Color is difficult to memorize, and a tool like the Renae Knapp "Personal Pro" Fan Deck can steer you toward making the right choices.

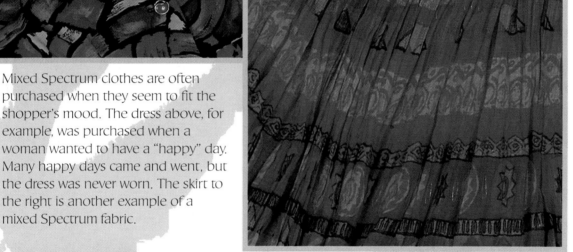

The Most Common Color Mistakes

The best word to describe the most common color mistakes is "emotional." Basing your purchasing decisions on emotion can mean several things. First of all, we often see someone looking fantastic in a certain color and we may say to ourselves, "I've got to have that." Or we'll ask, "Where did you get that?"—even though the color may not look very good on us at all. It is important to remember that each of us is uniquely color typed, and so are the colors that are best for us.

We can also be affected by Madison Avenue or Hollywood when making color choices solely based on fashion or trend. Going with fashion or trend is fine as long as the color choice is based on the science of the Blue Base/Yellow Base Color System. Otherwise, you begin to make a patchwork quilt out of your wardrobe and make-up colors.

Mixed Spectrum clothes are often purchased when they seem to fit the shopper's mood. The dress above, for example, was purchased when a woman wanted to have a "happy" day. Many happy days came and went, but the dress was never worn. The skirt to the right is another example of a mixed Spectrum fabric.

Be Cautious At Sales

Many sale items are on sale for the obvious reason: no one wanted them. Sometimes you can find a great buy, and it works perfectly with your pivotal colors. Most of the time, though, those items on sale are left over because neither Blue Base nor Yellow Base buyers wanted them. Anything that is mixed Spectrum creates a jarring effect on the eye. Even though the item could be extremely well made and a couture label, mixing the Spectrum in the fabric will give it a cheap, low-budget look.

Some shoppers may hold up a mixed Spectrum sale item and say, "I couldn't make it for that price." This brings up another point: never let price alone determine ownership of something. Even if the price is dirt cheap, the effects of wearing something in the opposite, or worse, mixed Spectrum, is not worth it.

In my seminars, I sometimes hold up two pieces of fabric given to me by clients. One is an $80 per yard mixed Spectrum silk fabric from Paris and the other is a $1 per yard harmonized Spectrum fabric. I ask the attendees which one they would consider to be the more expensive, and most choose the $1 swatch. Even though the other costs 80 times as much, the "richer" and more appealing fabric isn't mixed Spectrum like the expensive one.

But It Was A Gift

Does your mother or father ever buy you gifts that you can't tolerate? What about your friends, do they seem to have awful taste when it comes to gift giving? Research has shown that most of the time we buy for others based on our own color prejudices. We have a predisposition to purchase in our own Spectrum—even our own best colors. Consequently, others will do the same for us. If you know that someone always purchases items for you in your opposite Spectrum, you may want to get them a copy of this book as your next gift to them.

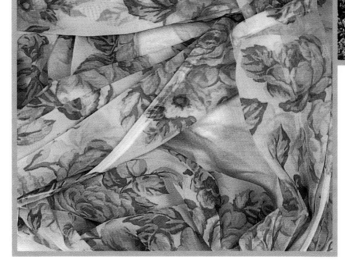

Scarves are especially prone to be mixed Spectrum because they are designed to make a statement. However, since they are worn next to the face, it is a very bad choice to ever wear a mixed Spectrum scarf. Look for fabrics that harmonize within one color Spectrum.

The Blue Base/Yellow Base Color System can be your greatest ally when you are shopping for just about anything. Whether you want a car, boat, new home, new suit, or new area of the country to move to, you will save enormous amounts of money and time by using this knowledge as a working tool in your life. You will also be a step ahead of the pack and never be a color victim again.

Sell Yourself With Color

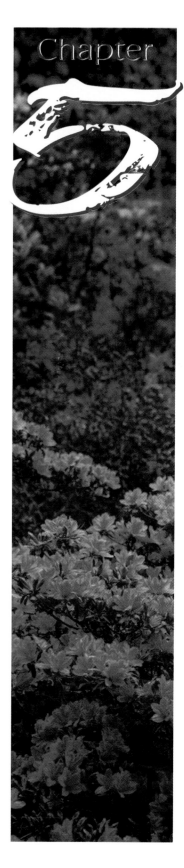

Here was a buyer's bargain. It hung securely from the side of the mountain, overlooking a spectacular valley below. The interior of the house was obviously of superior quality and displayed the finest craftsmanship—the home had no major flaws. It should have sold immediately. Instead, it sat on the market for several years. Finally, the desperate builder lowered his price to below cost.

The realtor who showed me the house admitted that it had become an obsession with him to sell the place. He couldn't understand why it wouldn't sell. Along with quality construction, it boasted a choice location. All the realtors had named it "the gingerbread house." It made no sense that this home was still on the market.

One look at the house and I knew instantly what was wrong. The exterior was a golden brown (Spectrum 2), and each window had pinkish-blue shutters (Spectrum 1). The trim was a Blue Base shade of blue and, for a grand finale, the focal points of the entire home were beautiful Blue Base green doors. It was a terrible, offensive, irritating mixed Spectrum mess. There was no harmony in the colors anywhere.

Inside the house, carpets, countertops, and tile floors were in Spectrum 1 colors, appliances in Spectrum 2. Everything about this house was perfect except for the color, and every potential buyer who went through it could hardly wait to leave.

All that was necessary to correct this mistake was some exterior paint and minor cosmetic changes, but without any knowledge of the Blue Base/Yellow Base Color System, no one had the vision or understanding to explain the problem. Instead of a rich, elegant, gracious appearance, the house had a tacky, cheap look. No one felt comfortable there.

Color Harmony Brings It Together

Another builder I know meticulously decorates his houses from one color group or the other, never mixing them. After several years of doing this, the results have been astounding. Even in times of recession and difficulty in the real estate business, his homes sell.

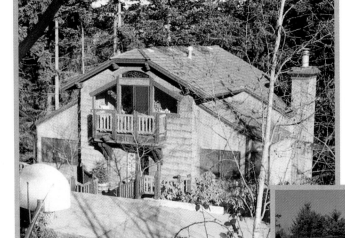

In the same manner as the "gingerbread house" (where everything on the surface looked right but nobody quite wanted it), you also present yourself to the world. How are you perceived at first glance? Are you someone who comes across as interesting and credible? Or does something seem just slightly out of place?

Roger Ailes, the former Presidential Image Advisor, has determined that we have seven seconds to present ourselves to others for the first time. In just seven seconds, others form a lasting opinion of us. The perception of that initial meeting may persist for many years, even if we prove ourselves to be otherwise.

Homes like these can be the best deals around, but often they won't sell because potential buyers feel that something is not quite right. They might not be able to name what's wrong, but the initial impact of color on the senses is often enough to end the sale.

Nixon-Kennedy Debate

The classic example of first impressions from American history was the Nixon-Kennedy 1960 presidential debate. Most of the American voters favored Nixon prior to the debate, yet most agreed that Kennedy had won the debate. In subsequent polls, most Americans not only thought that Kennedy looked better, but that he also understood the issues of the day better than Nixon. The only exceptions to that opinion came from those without televisions who had listened to the debate on the radio and did not actually view the candidates. Those radio listeners believed that it was a "no contest" victory for Nixon. The fact is that Nixon won the voters over verbally, while Kennedy won the nonverbal debate. Kennedy presented an image of competence that the American public believed from the moment they saw him.

You Are The Message

You can never simply say nothing. Everything you wear says something about you. A few years ago, I was asked to speak at a very large women's conference in Seattle where close to a thousand women would be present. I was asked to speak about self-esteem and how to feel good about yourself and who you are. I truly believe everyone can and should feel good about themselves and I was very excited to speak on this topic. After I had finished speaking, I went to a separate room to answer questions from attendees. It seemed like women were lined up for miles. One by one, I spoke to each individually about their personal coloring and how it impacted every area of their life.

As I spoke with each individual, I couldn't help noticing a woman standing slightly behind a pole that was close to me. She carefully listened to and observed each person as they spoke to me. She seemed to have immense interest in everything I said. After about an hour, I turned to her and said, "What would you like to ask me?" And then, as if on automatic pilot, I picked up one of my fabric swatches and said, "This would be a very dynamic color on you. You would look so beautiful." Not smiling, she looked at me through very sad eyes and said, "I would never do that. I don't want to stand out, I don't want anyone to notice me."

Then I glanced at her outfit, which was a very drab beige that I assume she wore on purpose to *not* attract attention. I looked at her and said, "That is never an option. No matter what you do, you are either telling the world 'I

Grace's whole appearance changed when she dressed in different Spectrums. When she wears Spectrum 2 colors (above), the shadows and lines on her face stand out and her skin looks pasty. When she wears her right Spectrum 1 colors (left) she looks young, vibrant, and confident.

like myself and I'm proud of who I am,' or 'I feel very negative about myself and this is who I am.'" Disappearing is not a choice for anyone. We are always perceived in one way or the other.

You can be conservative and still very confident looking. The style of clothes you choose is important, but wrong colors will overpower any style and leave a negative impression. Understanding the Blue Base/ Yellow Base Color System is the key to achieving positive results.

By now, you are getting in tune with the impact that color has on how you present yourself to the world. You are a part of the world. You truly are a part of nature and the great structure of this planet. In all of my research and travels around the globe, I have never once found anything in nature to be mixed Spectrum. I've never found a plant, animal or landscape that was mixed Spectrum. Even more exciting, I have never found a single human being who was mixed Spectrum. That's right—you are a perfect being, born into a Spectrum where everything about you harmonizes within that Spectrum!

When you present yourself wearing colors that go with what nature has given you, then you will immediately experience the power and attraction that comes from harnessing nature. You will sell yourself without speaking a word.

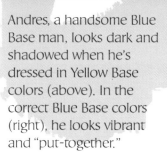

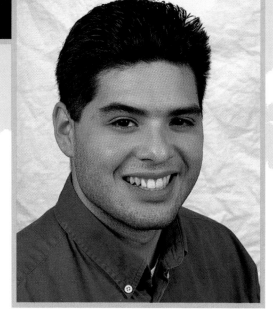

Andres, a handsome Blue Base man, looks dark and shadowed when he's dressed in Yellow Base colors (above). In the correct Blue Base colors (right), he looks vibrant and "put-together."

The only mistakes made in the world of color occur when humans mix Spectrums and create confusion with colors. Just like at a Las Vegas casino, we feel perplexed and jarred. Our eyes don't know where to land when Spectrums are mixed. We want to keep moving rather than relax.

While speaking to a large group of executives in Florida, I explained to them that people form an opinion about us in the first seven seconds after meeting us. They decide whether we are capable or not capable, smart or not so smart. We even get jobs or are rejected based on those first seven seconds. Since color is the first initial impact on our senses, the harmony or discord of the colors we dress in influence how people perceive us. We are literally rated in seven seconds, mostly based on color. People judge how well they like what they see and whether they are going to accept it.

After my talk, the president of the tobacco association came up to me and said, "I totally agree with what you said, Renae. We had a rather large position come open in our company. We interviewed for a month and finally filled the position with a person whose appearance was perfect and who seemed to be perfect for the job. Instantly, she turned out to be very bad. She just couldn't do the job. In a panic, we looked through the office and decided on a woman who had been with us for over 10 years. She had never been pro-moted because of her appearance. She just didn't look like she could do it. We gave her a chance and she turned out to be absolutely perfect. She is fabulous. What a lesson." He quickly added, "I, however, am the president of the company and can look any way I want. No one can fire me or mess with me." I had to agree that he had a valid point, but for those of us trying to compete in a very competitive world, we have to pay attention to color.

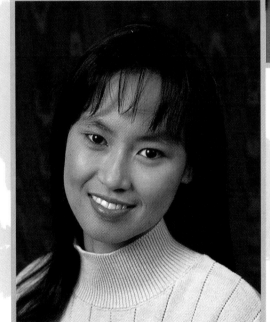

Sharon is a Blue Base woman. In the wrong Yellow Base colors (above) her skin tones seem brassy and the dark circles under her eyes are more pronounced. When she wears her correct Blue Base colors (left), she looks healthy, vibrant, and alert.

New Friends, Love, And Self-Esteem

Have you ever noticed how the sunset makes you feel? Or the peace that comes from being out in the countryside? One of my favorite pastimes is walking in nature and experiencing not only how perfectly the earth is put together, but also experiencing the beauty that is there.

My favorite definition of beauty is "a strong emotional response to a high degree of attraction." That simple definition sums it up for me. I always experience that strong emotional response when I look at our beautiful natural world. That is one reason why my company contributes to organizations—worldwide—that are dedicated to keeping nature beautiful and preserving it for our grandchildren.

Have you ever looked at anything in nature and experienced a strong emotional response? How about when you looked at another human? Isn't that called love at first sight? Believe it or not, my research has proven that we generally will attract and be attracted to those in our same Spectrum.

In the world of color, "likes" do attract. This generally works out best because you will agree on important purchasing decisions, where to live, and other major decisions much more readily with someone of your own color Spectrum.

The only time someone is unattractive to either Spectrum is when they are dressed in mixed Spectrum clothing or make-up. Our innate sense and craving for harmony and balance runs deep and influences our thinking. We are making countless unconscious decisions and judgments about life based on color. Nothing can be equal to the inner beauty of human beings, but until we get to know someone and the inner self, we will base our decisions on color first and form second. That's right: we see color in anything first and then notice the specific form or details second.

Recent tests conducted at UCLA have proven that beauty and harmony are innate desires, not ideals that are learned or taught. Researchers took a 15-day old infant to a dark room and showed the child two images— one of a woman with mixed Spectrum make-up and unbalanced proportions, and the other woman having correct Spectrum make-up and balanced proportions. The infant kept looking over at the woman with correct color and proportion. This happened even when its head was directed back to the other image.

We are all attracted to those who appear to "have it all together." It is not difficult to look totally together when you follow the simple science of the Blue Base/Yellow Base Color System. By putting yourself together in your own color Spectrum, you will look pulled together and will be amazed at the response others have toward your appearance.

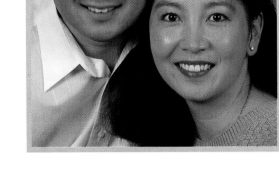

Scott and Lori, both attractive Blue Base adults, look vibrant and alive (bottom) when in their correct colors. You can see the difference between the wrong colors (top) and right colors (middle and bottom). Their three children could be either Blue Base or Yellow Base. Most likely, at least two of them will be Blue Base, though, as color is genetic.

Can Blind People See Color?

One day, I received a call from a blind woman. She said she was a psychiatrist with the University of Washington who not only taught but also had a thriving practice with many patients. She had just had her "colors done," and was typed into a season. Unfortunately, she just wasn't happy with the colors she had been given. She didn't think that it felt right. She had been given my name as a valid source to discover her true colors, using a scientifically proven method. She went on to say, "It is important to me, especially because I am blind, that people don't look at me and feel sorry for me. I want them to just feel comfortable around me and perceive my professionalism and focus on what I do." I spoke with her for a while, and we set a time for the appointment.

I have to admit that my brain was going really fast, trying to understand what she had just said. This threw a whole new light into having one's colors done. I read and studied all of the research on blind people and color. I knew that they could feel the color's energy, because each color has its own electromagnetic wavelength which strikes the cones and rods behind the eyes and vibrates them at a different rate. I could also understand the powerful impact that colors, used incorrectly, could have on her patients' perception of her. A mixed Spectrum creates a feeling of confusion and misunderstanding. This, coupled with her being blind, could be very negative and even harmful to her practice. I was very excited to explore all aspects of the system with a blind person. It was a wonderful opportunity for me to learn more. However, I was extremely anxious as to how this would all play out when she was actually sitting in front of me at the Renae Knapp Color Institute Salon.

The appointment time came, and due to her schedule, the psychiatrist arrived in the evening. Accompanying her was a beautiful dog that showed her every step of the way. She was brilliant and very much in control. She was confident and very excited to learn about color and how she could maximize its effects in her life. Seasonally, she had been placed in a season associated with Spectrum 2 colors. However, she was really a Spectrum 1, Blue Base person. As we started going through color swatches, I put the two blacks in front of her. I draped her with the Blue

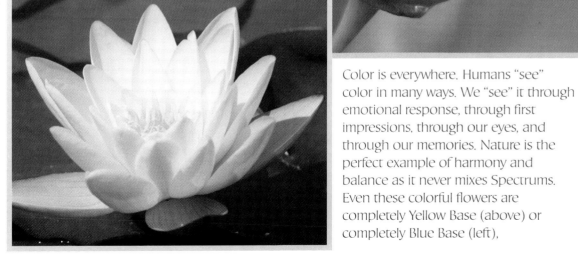

Color is everywhere. Humans "see" color in many ways. We "see" it through emotional response, through first impressions, through our eyes, and through our memories. Nature is the perfect example of harmony and balance as it never mixes Spectrums. Even these colorful flowers are completely Yellow Base (above) or completely Blue Base (left),

Base black, and then with the Yellow Base black. Instantly, it was apparent which Spectrum she was. As I told her, she grabbed the two blacks in her hands, one in each, and drew them close to her. Excitedly, she focused on the Blue Base black and said, "You're right! This one, this one is my black! Now I know why I didn't like that jacket in my closet. I knew something was wrong with the colors I had been given. Now I know why."

I was astounded to see this unfold in front of me. How exciting! She was literally feeling the energy of each black and could, in her fine tuned way, "see" the color. It was a wonderful experience for me to witness and confirmed what a powerful energy source color is. The system works for everyone, literally everyone, 100% of the time. It brings the same answer to the question *why*, and gives everyone the same confirmation of trusting ourselves, our inner knowledge, and the understanding of who we are.

Since my experience with the blind woman, I have even become a little impatient with those who say, "This is just not that important." Color harmony *is* important and should be understood by everyone! We all need to have a conscious awareness of color, appreciating what it means to us in daily life and taking notice of its tremendous influence on the planet. For those who complain that they can't see the difference between certain colors, remember, even blind people "see" color. We might even want to take a minute to enjoy color. If you need help identifying colors, one of the Renae Knapp Color Institute Salons can teach you how to distinguish between Blue Base and Yellow Base colors.

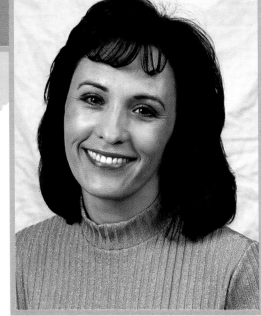

Maria, a striking Blue Base woman, looks tired and her skin looks faded when she wears Yellow Base colors (above). When she wears Blue Base colors (right), her skin looks healthy and she looks refreshed.

"We have all inherited a treasure of vast knowledge, but we must find a path to it. Beauty is one path to this treasure."

-Tarthang Tulku

The Ugliest Woman In The World

A customer of mine who worked for a large hotel chain referred a fellow employee to my institute. The employee, whom we shall call Beth, was very, very unattractive. In fact, she was so unattractive that she was kept hidden from everyone's view. The place she went to work each day was a very small room with no windows and no public access. She worked from a small table answering phones for the hotel. Although Beth had a beautiful voice, her self-esteem was nonexistent. She felt being hidden from the world was where she should be all her life. Her boss made it clear to her that she was to be very discreet in *how* she mingled in the hotel when she went on breaks or lunch. She was told to stay out of the main areas and not talk to anyone. She was completely handicapped and held hostage by her perception of how she looked, and how she really felt about herself. My customer, noticing this helpless person day after day while at work, finally decided to become proactive. She befriended Beth and then, in a kind way said, "You need to go see Renae." Beth was nervous, but my friend offered to go along with her the first time.

I have worked with thousands of men and women of all ethnicities, nationalities, and circumstances, but it was still a startling moment when Beth walked through my doors for the first time. I swallowed hard as I looked into the sad eyes of my unattractive new client. My mind was racing as I wondered how—and if—I could really help her. We talked for awhile, getting to know each other and feeling more comfortable with each other. She expressed her sad feelings about wanting to have a job where she could be with people and be seen, but at the moment she felt she couldn't even try. I looked into her eyes and said, "If you have a desire, I can give you the tools necessary to transform your inward and outward self." She very emphatically responded, "I have to do something. I can't go on like this, feeling such low self-esteem."

We started with the discovery of self and how we relate to the world through color

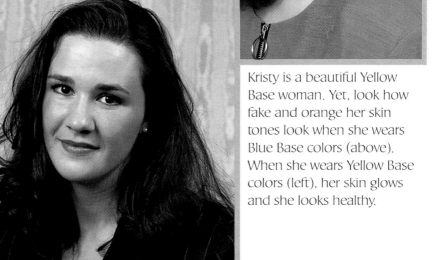

Kristy is a beautiful Yellow Base woman. Yet, look how fake and orange her skin tones look when she wears Blue Base colors (above). When she wears Yellow Base colors (left), her skin glows and she looks healthy.

science. Together, we looked at how color science's discovery of each person's unique individual coloring related to corresponding personality traits. She came completely alive when we did her personal colors, lines, and styles. After we had established the perfect tones, tints, and shades of her coloring, we created the perfect hair and cosmetics color palette. We carried her perfect colors into new wardrobe pieces and accessories. Everything flowed together in perfect harmony. She was understandably excited. This was more than a "make-over," this was information that would create a whole new lifestyle for her. Beth was learning valuable information that would literally change her whole life. It was all based on scientific research and validation, not just someone's opinion.

At the end of three weeks, Beth's whole countenance had changed. She stood taller, and her eyes were no longer sad. Instead, she projected excitement and enthusiasm for her new found knowledge of who she really was. She truly was ready to face the world at all costs. Her paradigm had completely changed.

When we receive new tools to help us, we are able to reexamine who we are in a clearer light. By heightening our self-awareness, we can be in control of who we are and how others perceive who we are. It is this knowledge of self that doesn't allow others to control us and our circumstances simply because we lack the tools to change their perception. Beth did go on to get a new job, new income, new friends, new clothes, and yes, even a new relationship!

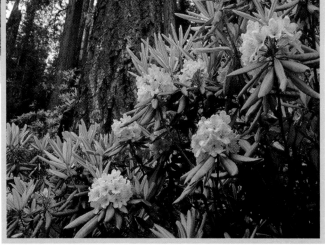

People everywhere feel drawn to nature, it calms them and makes them feel at peace. The perfect color harmony in nature plays a large role in the peacefulness of nature. We can use this knowledge to make ourselves exude a calm, peaceful aura through color harmony.

I challenge you to follow the principles laid out in this book. My desire is to see men and women everywhere achieve success and happiness in abundance. The information you have read is simple and easy to use. You already know most of it, I am just helping you focus the camera and see life through a clearer lens.

The 10 Most Frequently Asked Questions

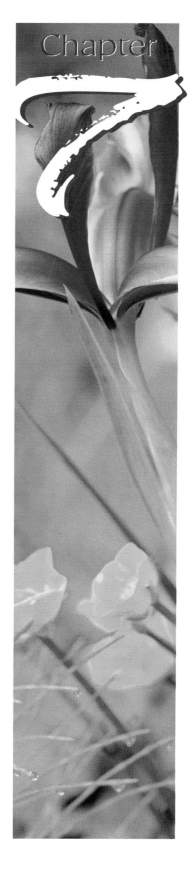

1. *How* do I determine the Spectrum of something with a Renae Knapp "Personal Pro" Fan Deck?

   Fan out your "Personal Pro" Fan Deck so that the whole range of Spectrum 1 colors and Spectrum 2 colors is visible. Then find the color swatches from each Spectrum that are closest to the color of the object in question and hold them up to the object. You will see very quickly which swatch best harmonizes with it. Remember, you don't need to get an exact match: it's harmony you're looking for. The color swatch from the appropriate Spectrum will seem to blend harmoniously with the object, whereas the color swatch from the opposite Spectrum will seem to stand out conspicuously.

2. *Won't the Spectrum of an object change, depending on its texture?*

   No, although, you will occasionally find that the colors of some textured objects may seem lighter or darker than the color swatch in your Renae Knapp "Personal Pro" Fan Deck. Some textured colors you are trying to match may be somewhat greyer in tone that the color swatch. Colors in both color groups can be greyed a bit without shifting from one color group to the other.

3. *Should Blue Base people wear only silver jewelry and Yellow Base people wear only gold?*

Absolutely not! Silver and gold are both metals and therefore do not absorb light—they only reflect it. Both will reflect your skin colors, so they can't help but look good. Go with the metal you prefer—and enjoy it. However, Spectrum 1 people with olive skin do look best in gold jewelry because of their skin pigmentation.

4. *If I have a lot of yellow in my skin, but I really like Spectrum 1 colors, does that mean I'm a mixed Spectrum person?*

No. There is no person who is "mixed Spectrum." Remember, there is a Spectrum 1 yellow. It has a bluish cast, which translates into olive skin tones. Sometimes Spectrum 1 people with this coloring label their skin a "sallow" yellow or "greenish" yellow, whereas Spectrum 2 people often label the yellow in their skin a "golden" yellow.

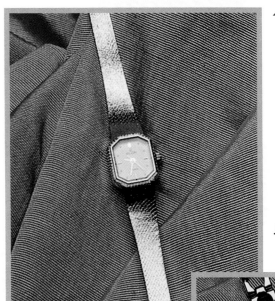

Jewelry that is gold or silver reflects the tones of whatever is around it. Both metals look good on both Spectrums. However, Yellow Base people often prefer brushed jewelry (above) while Blue Base people often prefer shiny jewelry (right).

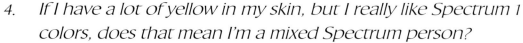

5. *If I have very pale skin with very little coloring, does that mean I'm a Spectrum 1 person?*

No. Lightness and darkness of skin color has no bearing on your Spectrum. The best clue to finding your Spectrum is to ask yourself which one you prefer and which one you love, and to look closely at your personal colors.

6. *If I want to highlight my mousy brown hair, what color should I ask for?*

Your calling your hair color "mousy brown" is a clue that you are probably a Spectrum 1 person.

These are the people who most often seek highlighting, frosting, or coloring to make up for the lack of natural highlights in their hair. Call the Renae Knapp Color Institute Salons at 1-888-395-9323 and we will put you in touch with a trained professional in your area who can help you with your questions.

7. *Am I all mixed up if my whole house is in Spectrum 2 colors but I'm a Spectrum 1 person?*

No. It sounds as though you're very normal. The Blue Base/Yellow Base Color System is a tool to help you recognize color harmony in both color groups. It is not meant to keep you from using both color groups in different aspects of your life. Living, dressing, and working in colors from only one color group would be boring. Don't mix the color groups on yourself and don't mix the color groups within specific rooms you decorate but, beyond that, enjoy!

8. *As I get older, will my Spectrum change?*

No, you will age in your Spectrum.

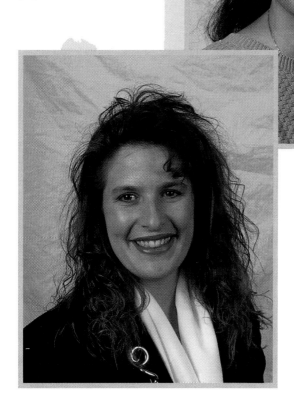

All three of these people are Blue Base. Thomas (top) has dark skin with definite plum highlights. Lori (middle) and Katherine (bottom) have rosy-pink highlights in their medium skin. Lightness or darkness of skin does not determine Spectrum.

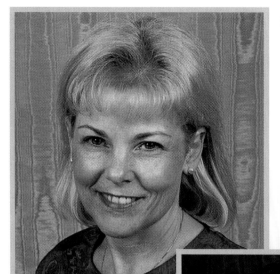

9. *Why do I see colors from both Spectrums combined in so many of the new fabrics?*

    Some textile designers try for a jarring look, or they feel that mixed-Spectrum fabrics are somehow more creative. In any case, this mixing of color groups violates all the principles of color harmony and is uncomfortable to live with for any length of time.

10. *If my spouse and I are both Yellow Base people, does that mean all of our children will also have Yellow Base coloring?*

    No. Skin, hair, and eye coloring are genetically determined. Although both my husband and I are Yellow Base people, only three of our five children have Yellow Base coloring. The others take after my mother (Blue Base) and my husband's father (Blue Base). Your Spectrum is totally linked with Mendel's law of heredity and genetic dominance. In the case of identical twins, they look alike, but each one has their own individual and unique characteristics, such as higher luminosity and lower luminosity.

These three people are all Yellow Base. Jane (top) has golden highlights in her fair skin. Francisco (middle) has very distinct peachy highlights in his medium skin, and Tina (bottom) like Jane, has definite golden accents in her dark skin.

Color Dynamics: Your Personal Color Profile

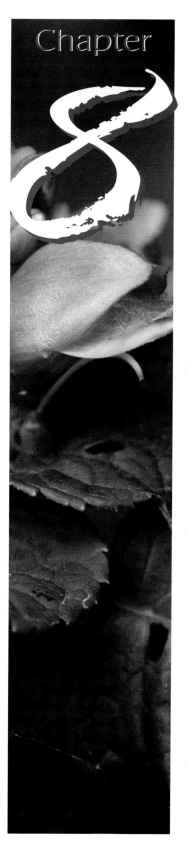

As mentioned previously, research has found that most people form a lasting opinion of someone within the first seven seconds of meeting him or her. Taking charge of your image and impact increases self esteem, closes deals, gets jobs, wins cases, makes new friends, and gives you credibility no matter what you do.

When your personal coloring harmonizes with your wardrobe and cosmetics, the message you send will be one of confidence and strength. By learning and understanding correct color science and theory and how it relates to personal coloring, you will immediately experience a more natural and radiant image. Correct personal color choices also eliminate costly mistakes by enabling you to buy only those items that work best for you.

The first step in discovering those colors that work best for you is to determine your personal color Spectrum and the colors within that Spectrum which are your personal best. The Renae Knapp Color Institute Salons have helped thousands of men and women worldwide use color to feel and look their very best. Take the following test as the first step to this process of discovering who you really are and how you personally fit into this scientific process.

Is My Personality Blue Base Or Yellow Base?

The test at the end of this chapter is to determine how your personality fits with your coloring. This has always been of major fascination and interest throughout the world. Yes, there are definite personality traits that correspond to an individual's coloring. Exciting scientific findings have been made on this subject. One such test was researched and developed by Keith Rogers, Ph.D., a brain domain theories expert from Brigham Young University. We met in the early 1990s and he became fascinated by the color science and my findings and information regarding the system.

Earlier testing has proven that genetically you are born into a Spectrum and you literally see the world through those eyes—Blue Base or Yellow Base. You love what is you and instinctively migrate toward your Spectrum.

If you are unsure about your personal color profile or want more help choosing colors, attend a Color Dynamics class offered at Renae Knapp Color Institute Salons. You will learn the following:

- Your personal colors—analyzed with samples to take home

- Your make-up in color harmony

- How to use your colors for maximum impact

- How to make educated purchasing decisions

Everyone needs to take this class at some time in his or her life. To find out when the next available class nearest you will be held, call 1-888-395-9323.

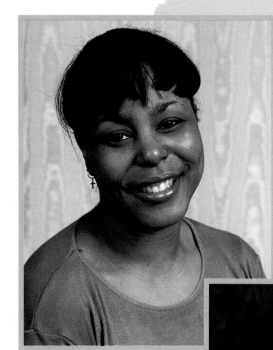

Dana, an attractive Blue Base woman, looks yellowed and tired when she wears Yellow Base colors (above). The dark circles under her eyes become more noticeable when she wears her wrong colors. When she wears her correct colors (right), she looks vibrant and healthy.

Color Personality Preference Questionnaire

Directions: Below are two columns of words or phrases in pairs. Simply choose from each pair the one that you prefer, and circle the symbol for that choice. There is no right or wrong answer. Simply read, choose, mark, and move on to the next. Stopping to figure it out will be a waste of time; go with your "gut-instinct."

1.	○	Shiny gold	●	Antique gold
2.	●	Pearls	○	Diamonds
3.	○	Russian sable fur	●	Canadian fox fur
4.	○	Designer jeans	●	Casual jeans
5.	●	Informal home decoration	○	Formal home decoration
6.	●	Working with my space	○	Working with other people
7.	●	Fieldstone	○	Marble
8.	○	Esthetics	●	Comfort
9.	●	Natural wood	○	Stained wood
10.	●	Unadorned	○	Ornate
11.	○	Campground with facilities	●	Wilderness with forest
12.	●	Barn wood	○	Polished oak
13.	●	Coarse weaves	○	Fine weaves
14.	○	Elegant	●	Rustic
15.	●	Informal dress	○	Formal dress
16.	○	Organizing things	●	Producing things
17.	●	The personal eye	○	The public eye
18.	○	Formal entertainment	●	Informal entertainment
19.	●	Smooth	○	Rough
20.	○	Patient, wait	●	Urgent, go
21.	●	Pewter	○	Silver
22.	○	Plan	●	Complete
23.	○	Management orientation	●	Results orientation
24.	●	Geography	○	History
25.	○	Spelling	●	Math
26.	●	Snorkeling	○	Sunbathing
27.	●	Casual	○	Hi-tech
28.	○	Directing	●	Coaching
29.	●	Situational tactics	○	Large scale strategies
30.	●	The practical	○	The ideal
31.	○	Silk	●	Wool

Totals: ○_____ ●_____   I chose: ❏ Spectrum 1 ❏ Spectrum 2

Now count the number of each you have circled—if you circled more ○ you are a more Blue Base personality, if you circled more ● you are a more Yellow Base personality.

Make-Up Tips That Get Results

As you experiment with the wonderful make-up colors that are found in your own color group, especially those reflected in your pivotal colors, remember that the application of cosmetics is an art form. You are creating an illusion and enhancing your features, just as you are when you select clothes for your wardrobe. Clothing and cosmetics in your color group bring your features and your own natural coloring into focus.

Make-up artistry is the art of applying color to facial surfaces—concave and convex—in such a way as to create balance, proportion, and definition to features or areas that would otherwise be imperfect or undefined. Light colors bring the focus forward while dark colors make the focus recede. The specific information that follows will help you blend color and technique more artfully, and thus enhance each area of your face.

A cover-up cream or concealer is used under the eyes to hide puffiness or circles. It is also used on blemishes and other facial imperfections to help hide them. Almost 90% of all concealers are Yellow Base. Blue Base people should wear a concealer with more of a pink tone so that it blends with the pink undertones of their skin.

Renae Knapp Body Care has produced an eye primer that works as a natural based cover-up for both Spectrums. There is also a perfect pressed powder (available in both Spectrums) that covers up blemishes.

Base Colors

The purpose of foundation is to even out skin tones and protect your skin from toxins in the environment. It can only even out skin tones if it is in the color group of the wearer. Foundation should be tested along the jawline and should never be more than half a shade darker than the natural skin tones. The shade is wrong if you have to apply it to the neck to get the skin tones to blend. The color is in the wrong color group if facial hairs look more pronounced. I took the guesswork out of the equation by making Renae Knapp Liquid Foundations in both Spectrums for absolute perfect cover—these are the only Blue Base/Yellow Base foundations on the market!

A conditioning duo-active pressed powder provides long lasting, even coverage, ensuring the skin surface a perfect smoothness while protecting it. The Renae Knapp Wet/Dry Foundations are the perfect product for this use. These, too, have been formulated in both Blue Base and Yellow Base Spectrums.

All but two foundations in the world contain some form of petroleum, which is very unhealthy for skin. Still, millions of people put pollutants on their most noticeable features everyday through their make-up. Renae Knapp Cosmetics are virtually the only cosmetics that do not contain these harmful substances.

A dusting of powder will give your make-up a finished, professional look and complete your work of art. Use a translucent or non-colored powder so as not to distort or detract from the colors in your facial palette. I have created a lavender powder for Blue Base people, and a peach powder for Yellow Base people, as well as other colors.

Eye Color

Brows are the frame for the eyes and should be as natural as possible. This means your brow pencil should be close in color to the hairs of your natural brow. Always brush brows with a soft brow brush (for instance, Renae Knapp Mini Brow Brush) for a natural look. I have also produced a soft line of Brush On Brow colors.

The term eye shadow itself denotes a color that should literally be a shadow of your own eye color. Shadows in your color group will highlight your eyes and cause them to look more radiant. Shadows in your opposite color group will conflict with your skin tones.

Powdered shadows (like Renae Knapp Eye Shadows) work best. They are easier to apply, and they stay where you want them to. In selecting eye shadow colors, remember our discussion in Chapter 3 where we pointed out that brown-eyed people, for example, do not just have brown eyes but rather brown with plums, blues, or purples around the iris. That's why certain plums and blues look so striking on them and complement their eyes. So, look for all the colors in your eyes (not the colors in your clothes,) and work with them in choosing eye shadow colors.

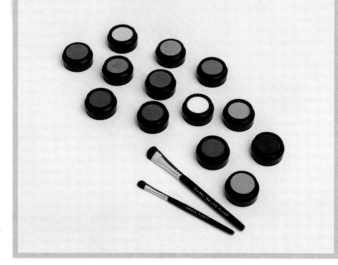

The colors around the iris are excellent guides to use in selecting eyeliner color. However, charcoal-grey and dark brown are basic colors that work well for most people.

People with deep set eyes should be very careful about wearing eyeliner. It tends to push the eyes further back into the head instead of

Renae Knapp Cosmetics are the only Blue Base and yellow base eye shadows available. It is vital that you use the correct eye shadows for your personal coloring to highlight your eyes. Using your wrong Spectrum colors creates a jarring or "made-up" look.

giving the eyes depth and definition. If you have deep set eyes and want to wear eyeliner, wear it under the bottom lash line only.

In selecting mascara color, be guided by your own color preference. I recommend a deep navy or blue mascara, because it's a wonderful color for people in both color groups. Blue colors make the whites of the eyes look whiter, thus setting off the actual eye color.

Yellow Base people should never wear jet black mascara. It's too harsh. My make-up line has a wonderful Yellow Base charcoal black, as well as jet black for Blue Base eyes.

Lips And Cheeks

Lipstick gives polish and finish to your look. If it's in your color group, lipstick also balances the face and helps avoid a top-heavy look by adding color to the bottom of the face. If your lipstick is in the wrong color group, you'll look out of proportion—"all mouth."

If you have a lot of depth in your natural coloring, don't be afraid of depth in your lip color. A lipstick that's too light will not bring all your coloring together into a glowing facial harmony.

Blusher is applied to the face to give color and accent to the cheekbones. Your blush color should harmonize with the undertones in your cheeks. Use a light hand in applying it; heavy blush color creates an overly made-up look. A good trick is to blend powdered blusher with translucent powder to soften the effect and then apply it with a wedge-shaped sponge.

You already know that your make-up should not clash with your clothes. Now you know that it is vital that your make-up not clash with your skin tones or your other make-up. Lip and cheek colors are often the most predominant colors you'll wear. It is vital that these colors not only be in your Spectrum, but that they be your best colors.

Blusher is a perfect example of color's ability to accentuate or diminish concave and convex surfaces, and to bring forward features or help them recede. Use a darker shade blush in the same color family as your main blush color to contour and sculpt the face. Place it below the main blush color, and blend them. This will give the under part of the cheekbones a recessed look.

Never choose a blush color with too high a luminosity level for your natural coloring. Blushers can be matte or frosted, but matte colors work best for most people. Use only matte for the contour color (try

Renae Knapp Conditioning Blush). Avoid cream blusher. It is more difficult to apply accurately, is easily absorbed by the skin, and does not work well on problem skin.

Nail Polish

Since polish is applied to nails, which are part of your fingers and hands, its color should be selected to harmonize with the skin tones of your hands, not those of your face. Frequently, I see women wearing the wrong color lipstick or make-up, but they always seem to have nail polish in their correct color group. I think that's because they see their hands constantly as they go through the day, while their face is not as visible to them. Renae Knapp Cosmetics have both Blue Base and Yellow Base nail colors available to help you look your best.

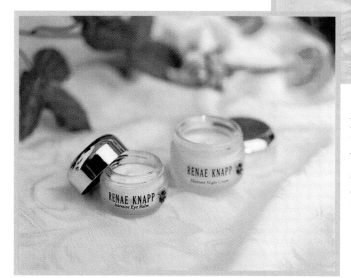

For information on purchasing products from the Renae Knapp Body Care and Cosmetics Collection call: 1-888-395-9323. (Refer to Appendix E for a complete product listing.)

Caring for yourself takes so little time, yet it affects you for a lifetime. Your face will be with you forever, and is what others see the most and you see the least. It is important that you care for your skin and apply the right make-up wisely.

What People Are Saying

Following are a few excerpts from some of the letters received by the Renae Knapp Color Institute Salons. They are included to show you how Renae Knapp Color Institute Salons are helping people every day.

Carol Norbeck, Vision Industry Council Of America

Thank you for teaching me the principles of the Blue Base/Yellow Base Color System. They have not only been the basis of eyewear fitting at Optical Illusions but, because of you, they have become the standard for the Envision Yourself program with the Vision Industry Council of America (VICA). Your continued support and especially your enthusiasm have always been an inspiration to me and other eyecare professionals.

The Blue Base/Yellow Base Color System, and the ability to determine the client's color base, is as integral a part of eyewear fitting as taking a PD or a seg height. The Blue Base/Yellow Base Color System, Facial Balance, Life-style Analysis, and Prescription are the four principles of Envision Yourself. The program is designed after the seminars that you and I developed back in 1980. Your ideas have been a continuing asset to me and to the optical industry.

Diane

Early in my government career, and before I met Renae and learned the color system, I wore jeans to work on a regular basis. Although my supervisor suggested that wearing jeans would not be the best for my advancement in the organization, I was confident that I would never "meet the *big* boss." One day, my supervisor called a group meeting—not unusual in our business. I recall sitting in the back of the room, trying to be "inconspicuous" in my jeans. As the meeting continued, the *big* boss joined us. The supervisor introduced him and the reason why she invited him—to present a Special Act Award to a member of her group. As the citation was read it was apparent that I was to be the recipient. That day I did meet the big boss—in my jeans.

Shortly after this, I had the opportunity to meet Renae and was introduced to the color system. The most powerful message she presented was the impact that color has. I am a Blue Base individual, and blue jeans were not the way to impress my boss. I now have confidence wearing the colors that enhance me when making presentations to senior government officials. I know that what I am wearing is not a distraction to the message that I am presenting.

I have also been wearing Renae Knapp Cosmetics. The quality of the product is far superior to any product that I have used before. At the end of my long days I look as fresh as I did when I first applied it! I have received many comments on the look that it achieves.

Oh, by the way, my career has been very successful. Since that first jeans experience, I have received five promotions.

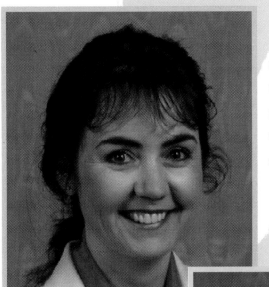

Lisa's whole appearance changes when she dresses in different Spectrums. When she wears Spectrum 2 colors (above), the shadows and lines on her face stand out and her skin looks pasty. When she wears her right Spectrum 1 colors (right) she looks young, vibrant, and confident.

Julie

When I first went to see Renae Knapp for my personal coloring and make-up, I knew I had found something fabulous. What I did not know, then, was how dramatically my life would change and how positively my life would be influenced. I have never looked at anything the same since. I am a believer in the Blue Base/Yellow Base Color System. The phenomenal results of using the Blue Base/Yellow Base Color System and the quality of Renae Knapp Body Care and Cosmetics simply sell themselves.

Ashley

Several years ago, I was introduced to the Blue Base/Yellow Base Color System and the significant effort it has on so many aspects of my life. I caught on right away and couldn't help but be amazed as well as intrigued. I wanted to know more. To me, Renae Knapp is nothing less than miraculous! I can't begin to express my happiness—thank you Renae!

Louise

I get compliments on how great I look when I wear the Renae Knapp Cosmetics in my color Spectrum. I am a redhead and tend to have dry skin and chapped lips. Since I have used Renae's products, I have never had chapped lips or dry skin! Plus, I used to have sun allergies and since wearing the Renae Knapp foundation, I don't!

Clay

We could not agree on how to decorate our new home. My wife and I had different color preferences and there seemed to be no common ground. When we understood the Blue Base/Yellow Base Color System, we were able to pull our home together in one week. It literally saved our marriage. Thank you for that valuable information.

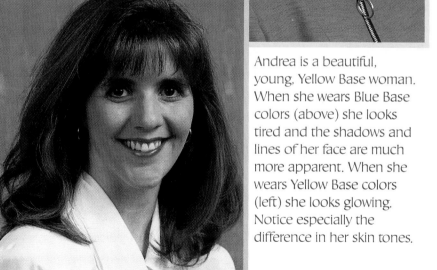

Andrea is a beautiful, young, Yellow Base woman. When she wears Blue Base colors (above) she looks tired and the shadows and lines of her face are much more apparent. When she wears Yellow Base colors (left) she looks glowing. Notice especially the difference in her skin tones.

Katherine

I have tried for many years to find make-up that would hide the birthmark on my face. I had no success. If I did find make-up that matched my skin tone, I would have to "cake" it on to cover it up. Renae Knapp Cosmetics are great! The foundation blends so well with my natural skin tones that my birthmark appears to have vanished. I have also found the make-up to be very comfortable to wear—not thick, greasy, and heavy feeling. I would recommend this make-up to anyone searching for a skin product to use on their birthmarks, scars, or blemishes.

Katherine is a perfect example of how vital matching skin tones is. The photo above is her birthmark with no make-up on it. The bottom photo is the birthmark with the wrong, Yellow Base make-up on. The middle photo is the birthmark with Katherine's correct Blue Base colors on. Notice how the birthmark virtually disappears when it is blended with the correct base color.

Rosemarie

Thanks so much! I sincerely mean thanks. I feel so good. Saturday my son said to me, "Mom, you look like a fashion plate, you looked very sharp yesterday, too." Coming from him, that was terrific! I needed that!

Kay

I would say that this is the wisest investment I've ever made. I'm having fun with the new me!

Wendy

I can't imagine my life without the Renae Knapp Blue Base/Yellow Base Color System! When I was first exposed to the Renae Knapp Color Institute Salons, I was fresh out of high school. As an insecure 18 year old, I was floundering in choices about colleges and careers, not to mention how to shop and how to put on make-up. What I knew about clothes and make-up came from what looked good on someone else, and trying to copy that. That all changed after I understood and started applying the Blue Base/Yellow Base Color System. My life revolves around being a Blue Base person. My favorite color is plum! I just love it when people say, "Oh, that plum color looks so good on you!"

Lorinda

Being in the optical business I worked with many color systems as clients came in to select frames. Until I met Renae and learned the Blue Base/Yellow Base Color System, it was all very confusing for both the client and me. I was a frame buyer for eight stores in the Pacific Northwest. After learning the system, I was able to control my inventory and save considerable money for my company. On a personal level, Renae has given me the confidence needed in a very competitive business to know that I am good at what I do.

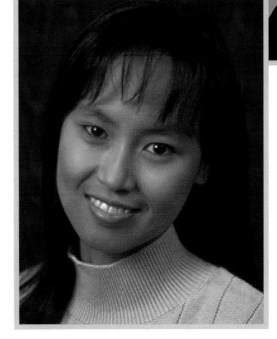

Correct colors and color harmony make the difference between people looking just okay and looking spectacular. Keiko (above) and Sharon (left) demonstrate this to be true.

Sally

I was first introduced to Renae Knapp and the Blue Base/Yellow Base Color System in May of 1997. With my experience in other color philosophies, I could see that there was more to know. I was very interested. Immediately, I had my personal colors analyzed and loved the results. With the other theories I never felt satisfied or complete. I could envision the benefits of incorporating the science into my cabinet business. Renae has assisted me in keying and creating new stains for cabinets and my customers are incredibly excited.

I have used the Renae Knapp Body Care line for months and my skin feels healthy and wonderful. Also, by using the cosmetics in my Blue Base colors, I feel completely dressed. The one aspect I love the very most about this is that I can introduce a color system that is scientifically proven to be 100% accurate and it's changing peoples lives around the world!!!! Thank you, Renae.

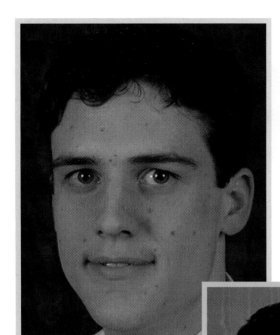

Aaron, a handsome Yellow Base man, has freckled skin. When he wears Blue Base colors (above), his freckles and moles stand out. They are more understated when he wears his correct colors (right).

Dan

We needed colors that would work to promote mental health in our center for abused women. We called the Renae Knapp Color Institute Salons for help. The colors chosen have been extremely positive. The atmosphere is calming and yet happy feeling. This is important since it rains constantly in Seattle. The results through color have been wonderful.

Cheri

I recently purchased a new home. After moving in I found there were some rooms that I felt instantly at home in and others that looked "off." All the furnishings were a similar style. It wasn't until I learned the Blue Base/Yellow Base Color System and how to determine color harmony that I knew why. I saved a lot of money and stress by changing one or two items in the room instead of all the furnishings. Now my home feels harmonious and the way I dreamed a home should be. Thank you, Renae.

Continuing Your Color Education

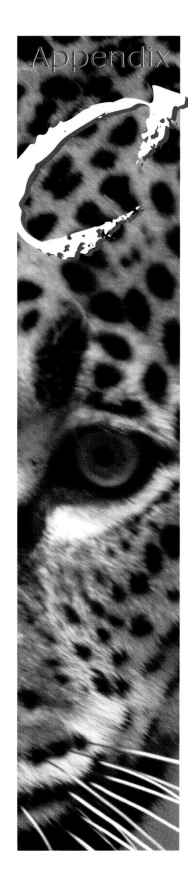

Throughout this book, I have presented you with a new way of looking at the world of color. I have given you some easy-to-follow guidelines to make color a working tool in your life. In order to continue learning what a difference the Blue Base/Yellow Base Color System can have on your daily life, visit one of the Renae Knapp Color Institute Salons worldwide.

On the following page is a listing of Renae Knapp Color Institute Salon locations. Call the one nearest you today to schedule a haircutting or haircoloring appointment, or to register for the next available color class.

Remember, Renae Knapp Color Institute Salons are the only valid source for Blue Base/Yellow Base Color System products and services. Salons are opening constantly; new breakthroughs and ideas are discovered everyday. For questions regarding services, products, and education, or for the most up to the minute information regarding the location of new salons, or if your are a professional stylist and would I like to know about employment opportunities, call us at 1-888-395-9323 or visit us at www.livingincolor.com.

Location	Executive Director	Phone
Billings, Montana	Lynette Michael	406-259-9540
Chicago, Illinois	Abi Carmen	847-755-1500
Irvine, California	Barry Knapp	949-251-1445
Las Vegas, Nevada (East)	Mary Wellmon/Bonnie Knell	702-968-8025
Las Vegas, Nevada (West)	Sally Cox	702-968-8025
Salt Lake City, Utah	Bonnie Knell/Marie Olsen	435-674-2988
Seattle, Washington	Julie Mitchell	206-244-9770
St. George, Utah	Bonnie Knell/Marie Olsen	435-674-2988

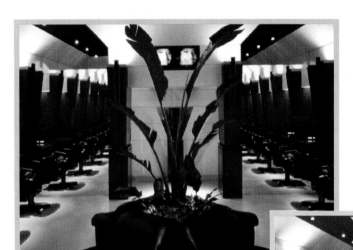

Renae Knapp Color Institute Salons are currently being opened around the world. The Salons look like these photos—Yellow Base (above) and Blue Base (right).

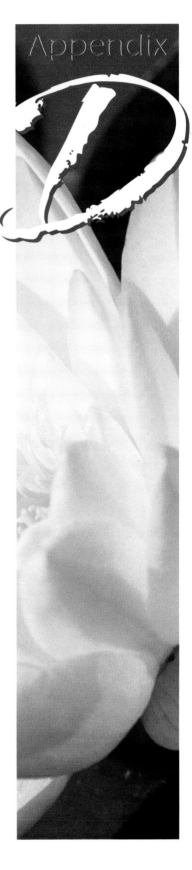

Warning!

Do Not Read This Section Unless You Value Your Skin

If you would like to know how nearly all skin and body care products in the world are literally costing men and women their lives—adding years before their time and sapping them of vital energy and stamina—this is going to be the most interesting message you will ever read.

Here is why: back in the 1930s, skin was thought to be impermeable and a truly protective coating. By the 1960s, skin was viewed as permeable and researchers demonstrated that some pesticides and lead in paint could enter the body through the skin. By the 1980s, molecular biologists began experimenting with the skin as a reactive, dynamic organ. This was when transdermal patches such as nicotine, heart, and motion sickness patches that delivered drugs into the body through the skin were developed.

By the 1990s, cosmetics, hair care, and body care were viewed by many scientists (and even the American Medical Association) as transmitters of toxins and coal tars into the body through the skin. Cancers of every type, allergies, toxic poisonings, weak immunities, along with psychological and depression problems, have developed and progressed through the personal care products used by men and women. And, the biggest discovery is that most of these effects are caused by the ingredients being derived from *petroleum waste and chemicals found in 98% of all soaps, shampoos, cleansers, and cosmetics!*

So why do the FDA and the chemists formulating these products allow these nasty ingredients into personal care products? First of all, petroleum waste is a potentially big problem. The mere cost of meeting environmental waste laws is enormous for oil refineries. That is why every major oil company has turned their toxic waste problem into a tremendous profit center (a business practice started by the Rockefellers decades ago). Their albatross has become the daily body care and cosmetics industry for billions of people worldwide.

Have you ever used Vaseline, petroleum jelly, or mineral oil? In truth, only a mere 3% of the personal care brands worldwide even claim to use "All Natural" ingredients. In a recent study of the 100 top-selling "natural" personal care brands, all of them, with one exception, used some of the same harmful petroleum and chemical preservatives as the other brands, but simply added some herbs or vitamins to the formula.

Simply adding some herbs and vitamins on top of the toxic chemicals is a bit like spooning whipping cream on top of a mud pie—the effects of the petroleum preservatives and chemicals are overwhelming!

Think about what this means: even though the products that you are using contain natural ingredients and have a nice smell to them. *They are still likely to have lots of horrible stuff in them when you wash your face or body with them!*

When I discovered this, I was horrified! I, along with millions of Americans, had been poisoning myself daily! In an effort to stop damaging my skin and my health, I decided to create my own personal care products. This was the beginning of the Renae Knapp Personal Care and Cosmetics lines.

My products truly are all natural. They are packed with herbs and vitamins. But more important, they have no harmful toxins or chemicals.

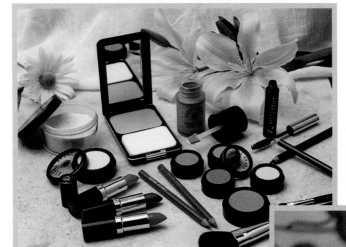

Renae Knapp Personal Care and Cosmetics are available at Renae Knapp Color Institute Salons across the world. For a free catalog of available products and to locate a Renae Knapp Color Institute Salon near you, call 1-888-395-9323 today!

Renae Knapp Product Collection

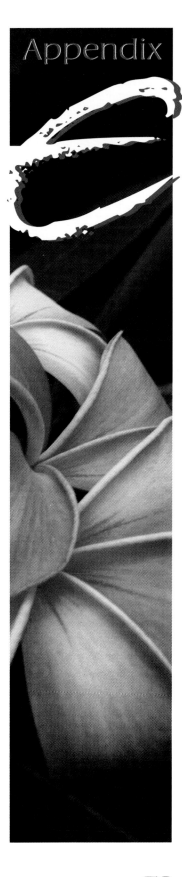

Dear Customer:

Welcome to the Renae Knapp cosmetic collection! For over 30 years now, I have conducted extensive research in applying the Blue Base/Yellow Base color science to high quality make-up and skin care. Continuing the research initiated by color scientist Robert Dorr, I have developed a premier make-up collection providing exacting colors for your individual skin tones and color Spectrum. Whether you have a blue undertone or yellow undertone, I am confident that you will find your perfect look with Renae Knapp Body Care Products and Cosmetics.

A trained Renae Knapp Associate will be happy to help you select your best colors and skin care products.

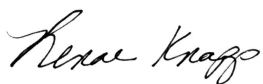

Balancing Foundations

Spectrum 1

#1001   Satin Porcelain (fair)
#1002   Rose Beige (medium)
#1003   Natural Beige (tan)

Spectrum 2

#2001   Almond Beige (light golden)
#2002   Natural Porcelain (medium beige)
#2003   Deep Beige (tan)

This oil free formula, enriched with anti-aging ingredient Rosemary and a Ceramide complex, protects skin from the environment while blending perfectly with your skin tones for a perfectly natural look. Exclusive natural sunscreen formula protects skin all day. Although not pictured, Renae Knapp Liquid Foundations are also available for dark skin tones.

Wet/Dry Foundations

Spectrum 1
#1050 Soft Beige (light)
#1051 Rose Bisque (tan)

Spectrum 2
#2050 Cream Beige (light)
#2051 Tender Beige (tan)

Oil and fragrance free, the exclusive conditioning formula of duo-active pressed powder, gives long lasting even coverage. Wet/Dry Foundation ensures the skin surface a perfect smoothness when applied over Renae Knapp Balancing Foundation. Used under liquid foundation, it hides imperfections, making a perfect concealer.

Loose Powders

Colors

#0080 All Natural (translucent)
#1080 Radiant Lavender (Blue Base)
#2080 Radiant Peach (Yellow Base)

Renae Knapp's Loose Powder, perfect for all skin types, reduces shine while setting make-up colors and keeping them looking fresh. The fine texture and natural ingredients give a luxurious and silky feel.

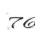

Blushes

Spectrum 1

#1201 Berry Wine
#1202 Cranberry
#1204 Cherry Plum
#1205 Watermelon

Spectrum 2

#2201 Cajun
#2202 Adobe
#2203 Valencia
#2204 Santa Fe
#2205 Pink Coral

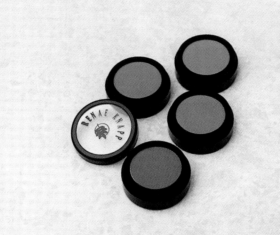

The Renae Knapp blush colors collection has been carefully designed and selected for individual skin tones and pigmentations which occur most often. The customized colors present a perfect match for skin tones of either Spectrum 1 or Spectrum 2. Active levels of Dimethicone and Squalane (olive oil) provide conditioning and protection.

Eyeshadows

Spectrum 1		Spectrum 2	
#1101	Amethyst	#2101	Eggplant
#1102	Wisteria	#2102	Violet
#1103	Sophia Pink	#2103	Rosequartz
#1104	Tea Rose	#2104	Sandstone
#1105	Mahogany	#2105	Terra Cotta
#1106	Rosewood	#2106	Java
#1107	Emerald	#2107	Sage
#1109	Pebble	#2108	Victoria Blue
#1110	Alabaster	#2109	French Vanilla
#1111	Plum	#2110	Slate
#1112	Pink Topaz	#2111	Indigo
#1113	Pink Suede		
#1114	Iris		

Renae Knapp eliminates the guesswork in finding the right colors with an exclusive collection of customized eyeshadow shades available in Spectrum 1 and Spectrum 2 colors. Because shades are based on correct tones found in human pigment, these eyeshadows give a naturally beautiful setting to the eye resulting in color that's never overpowering.

Eye Pencils And Cake Liners

Pencil Eyeliners:		Cake Eyeliner	
#0601	Storm	#1250	Coal Black
#0602	Denim		(Blue Base)
#0603	Raven	#2250	Muted Black
#0604	Evergreen		(Yellow Base)
#0605	Coffee		
#0606	Caribbean		
#0609	Mocha		
#0610	Grape		
#0611	Teal		
#0613	Blueberry		

The Eye Pencils are designed in Germany exclusively for Renae Knapp. These pencils provide lasting definition to eyes in either color Spectrums. The Cake Eyeliners go on smoothly to define and clarify the eye. An exclusive formula is gentle to the delicate eye area.

Brush On Brows

Colors

#0450 Soft Charcoal
#0451 Sable
#0452 Taupe

Designed to soften and fill the important and often overlooked eyebrow area, this unique formula gives just the right amount of color for defining and framing the eye color while conditioning the eyebrows.

Mascaras

Spectrums 1

#1402   Royal Blue
#1410   Black Onyx

Spectrum 2

#2401   Whisper Black
#2403   Navy

Conditioners in Renae Knapp Mascaras build and lengthen lashes while giving them essential nutrients. The result is fuller, healthier lashes. A thick brush makes applying the mascara simply and easy. These mascaras come in Spectrum 1 and Spectrum 2 colors.

Lipsticks

Spectrum 1

#1341 Flame
#1342 Orchid
#1343 Wine
#1344 Fuchsia
#1345 Romance
#1346 Soft Mauve
#1347 Milan

Spectrum 2

#2342 Strawberry Daiquiri
#2343 Iced Tea
#2344 French Poppy
#2345 Cherry
#2346 Frosted Copper

Emulsifying lip colors, with a natural SPF, protect lips while maintaining radiant color in either Blue Base or Yellow Base shades. Each color is heat sealed at production to ensure lasting freshness and firmness.

Lip Liner Pencils

Spectrum 1

#1520 Azalea
#1523 Blossom
#1525 Damask Rose
#1527 Ruby Red
#1529 Valentine

Spectrum 2

#2507 Sunset
#2524 Dune

The ultimate in lining and defining, Renae Knapp Lip Liners enhance and contour any lip color from pinks to bronze tones. These pencils are perfect for lining or filling in lips.

Professional Brushes

Brushes

#4009 Complete Set of Brushes
#4001 Mini Duster (Blush)
#4002 Powder Brush
#4003 Brow/Lash Groomer
#4004 Eyeliner
#4005 Chisel Fluff Deluxe
#4006 Small Fluff
#4007 Mini Brow
#4008 Angle Detail

Renae Knapp make-up brushes were designed personally by Renae Knapp for professional make-up artists. Now you, too, can take advantage of these pure sable, professional quality make-up brushes as your personal tools for designing your perfect face.

Essential Skin Care

For Normal To Oily Skin
#3001 Essential Deep Cleanser
#3002 Purifying Facial Toner

For Normal To Dry Skin
#3101 Gentle Orange Cleanser
#3102 Refreshing Aloe Toner

For All Skin Types
#3201 Herbal Vitamin Mist (1 oz.)
#3202 Herbal Vitamin Mist (6 oz.)
#3203 Nutrient Night cream
#3204 Intensive Eye Balm
#3208 Rejuvenating Moisturizer
#3209 Gentle Eye Makeup
        Remover
#0410 Oil Control Sea Kelp
        Powder
#0411 Eyeshadow Primer

At Renae Knapp Color Institute Salons, beautiful skin tones and make-up begin with healthy skin. Whether your skin is dry, normal, or oily, Renae Knapp provides a fast, intelligent, and simple, natural solution to cleansing and nourishing. Renae Knapp skin care delivers the finest, most technologically advanced products you will find anywhere.

Hair And Body Collection

For Both Spectrums

Purifying Shampoo
Purifying Conditioner
Shape Styling Creme
Fast Hold Spray
Rejuvenating Body Lotion
Purifying Body Cleanser

Renae Knapp Purifying Hair and Body Collection, like the rest of the collection, are formulated to provide a simple, natural solution to cleansing and nourishing the body as well as the hair.

For More Information

To find out more about other color products or services offered at Renae Knapp Color Institute Salons worldwide, or to schedule a free personal coloring consultation, contact your Renae Knapp Independent Associate. Call 1-888-395-9323, or visit us online at www.livingincolor.com today!

Renae Knapp Color Institute Salons are known for friendly and personal consultations that use technology to provide you with accurate color information and help you look your best.

Color And The Optical Industry

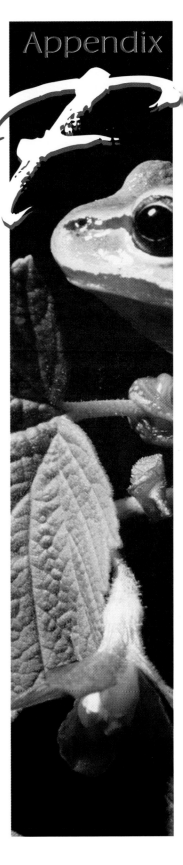

Manufacturers, eyecare providers, laboratories and all others involved in the delivery of quality eyecare and eyewear products enjoy the benefits of VICA's (Vision Industry Council of America), efforts. VICA is a not-for-profit trade association founded by a group of optical industry leaders.

VICA's mission statement, in part, is to:

1. Communicate the importance of eyecare and eyewear to target markets.

2. Improve the marketing skills of eyecare providers to help them prosper.

3. Provide forums for the exchange of industry information.

Also, included in this mission statement is a strong commitment to education.

The Blue Base/Yellow Base Color System color science is a major part of that education in the Optical Industry. Optical professionals using the system find a strong referral system because clients love how they look and feel in the correct Spectrum.

For more information on the Vision Industry Council of America (VICA) and the services provided please call 1-800-424-8422. To receive professional training and personal consultations regarding the optical industry, please call Carol Norbeck at (360) 898-4404.